PRIMITIVE BODILY COMMUNICATIONS
IN PSYCHOTHERAPY
Embodied Expressions of a Disembodied Psyche

PRIMITIVE BODILY COMMUNICATIONS
IN PSYCHOTHERAPY

Embodied Expressions of a Disembodied Psyche

Edited by Raffaella Hilty

KARNAC

KARNAC

First published in 2022 by Karnac Books, an imprint of Confer Ltd. London
www.confer.uk.com

Registered office:
Brody House, Strype Street, London E1 7LQ, UK

Copyright © Confer Ltd., 2022
Foreword © Susie Orbach, 2022

The right of the editor to be identified as the author of the editorial material, and of the authors for their individual chapters, has been asserted in accordance with sections 77 and 78 of the Copyright, Designs and Patents Act, 1988. All rights reserved. No part of this document may be reproduced or transmitted in any form or by any means, electronic, mechanical, photocopying, recording, or otherwise, without prior written permission of the copyright owners.

1 3 5 7 9 10 8 6 4 2

This is a work of nonfiction. Some names and identifying details may have been changed or omitted to, in part, protect the privacy of individuals.
Every effort has been made to trace the copyright holders and obtain permission to reproduce this material. If you have any queries or any information relating to text, images or rights holders, please contact the publisher.

British Library Cataloguing in Publication Data
A catalogue record for this book is available from the British Library.

ISBN: 978-1-913494-30-8 (paperback)
ISBN: 978-1-913494-31-5 (ebook)

Typeset by Bespoke Publishing Ltd.
Printed in the UK

FSC MIX Paper from responsible sources FSC® C011748

Contents

ABOUT THE AUTHORS		vii
ACKNOWLEDGEMENTS		xi
FOREWORD *by Susie Orbach*		xiii
USE OF TERMS		xvii
INTRODUCTION *by Raffaella Hilty*		xix

1. The spitting patient: speaking with sputum and free-associating with saliva
   Brett Kahr — 1

2. Working with primitive bodily communications in the context of unbearable trauma in non-verbal patients
   Valerie Sinason — 51

3. The sound of silence: working with people with an intellectual disability who self-harm
   David O'Driscoll — 63

4. Patients who smell: olfactory communication and the mephitic other
   Gabrielle Brown — 79

5. Body odour in a psychoanalytic treatment: bridge or drawbridge to a troubled past?
   Raffaella Hilty — 99

6. *In corpore inventitur*: embodied countertransference and the process of unconscious somatic communication
   Salvatore Martini — 119

7. Revisiting the entropic body: when the body is the canvas
   Tom Wooldridge — 141

8. When the psyche shreds and the body takes over   157
   William F. Cornell

9. Responding to trauma-based communication in psychotherapy   181
   Mark Linington

REFERENCES   199

INDEX   225

About the authors

Gabrielle Brown BPC, FPC, DipSW is a forensic psychotherapist at the Portman Clinic, Tavistock and Portman NHS Trust, London. *Psychoanalytic Thinking on the Unhoused Mind* was published by Routledge in 2019.

William F. Cornell, MA maintains an independent private practice of psychotherapy and consultation in Pittsburgh, PA. He teaches internationally with a primary focus on working with somatic processes and sexuality. Bill is a founding faculty member of the recently inaugurated Western Pennsylvania Community for Psychoanalytic Therapies. He is the author of *Explorations in Transactional Analysis: The Meech Lake Papers*; *Somatic Experience in Psychoanalysis and Psychotherapy: In the Expressive Language of the Living*; *Self-Examination in Psychoanalysis and Psychotherapy: Countertransference and Subjectivity in Clinical Practice*; *At the Interface of Transactional Analysis Psychoanalysis, and Body Psychotherapy: Theoretical and Clinical Perspectives*, and *Une Vie Pour Etre Soi*. He is a co-author and editor of *Into TA: A Comprehensive Textbook*, which has been translated into several languages. Bill has published numerous articles and book chapters, many of which have been translated into French, Italian, German, Portuguese, and Chinese. Bill edited and introduced books by James T. McLaughlin, Warren Poland, and Wilma Bucci. An editor of the *Transactional Analysis Journal* for fifteen years, he is now the editor of the Routledge book series, 'Innovations in Transactional Analysis'. Bill is a recipient of the Eric Berne Memorial Award and the European Association for Transactional Analysis Gold Medal in recognition of his writing.

Raffaella Hilty MA (Phil) is an attachment-based psychoanalytic psychotherapist with The Bowlby Centre. She has worked as an honorary psychotherapist within the NHS for a number of years, and she now works in private practice in London.

Professor Brett Kahr has worked in the mental health profession for more than 40 years. He is Senior Fellow at the Tavistock Institute of Medical Psychology in London and, also, Visiting Professor of Psychoanalysis and Mental Health at Regent's University London. A Consultant in Psychology to The Bowlby Centre and a Consultant Psychotherapist at The Balint Consultancy, he works with both individuals and couples in private practice in Central London. A trained historian as well as a clinician, he has recently become Honorary Director of Research at Freud Museum London, having served for many years on the museum's Board of Trustees. Kahr has maintained a long-standing interest in disability psychotherapy and, in collaboration with Dr. Patricia Frankish, Professor the Baroness Hollins [Sheila Hollins], and Dr. Valerie Sinason, he co-founded the Institute of Psychotherapy and Disability back in 1999. He has now become a Fellow of this organisation and continues to champion the provision of psychotherapy for severely and profoundly disabled adults and children.

He has authored sixteen books on a range of mental health topics, including the very first biography of Great Britain's leading psychoanalyst, *D.W. Winnicott: A Biographical Portrait*, which won the Gradiva Award for Biography in 1997, as well as *Sex and the Psyche*, the largest study on the role of trauma in the genesis of sexual fantasies, and, most recently, *Freud's Pandemics: Surviving Global War, Spanish Flu, and the Nazis*. His forthcoming book is entitled *How to Be Intimate with 15,000,000 Strangers: Musings on Media Psychoanalysis*. Kahr has also served as Series Editor of over 75 additional books on a range of topics, including couple and family psychoanalysis, forensic psychotherapy, and the history of psychoanalysis.

Mark Linington is an attachment-based psychoanalytic psychotherapist with The Bowlby Centre and the Clinic for Dissociative Studies in London. From 2013 to 2018 he was CEO at The Bowlby Centre, where he continues to work as a training therapist, clinical supervisor and teacher. He worked for 12 years in the NHS as a psychotherapist with children and adults with intellectual disabilities, who experienced complex trauma and abuse. He also worked as a psychotherapist for several years at a secondary school in London for young people with special needs, including autism, ADHD and other intellectual disabilities.

He has written a number of papers and book chapters about his clinical work and presented papers on attachment theory in clinical practice at a number of conferences, including in South Korea, Hong Kong and Paris. He is currently Clinical Director and CEO at the Clinic for Dissociative Studies, where he is a specialist consultant psychotherapist and clinical supervisor, working with people with a Dissociative Identity Disorder (DID). He works in private practice with children, adults and families and provides supervision to individuals and groups and training to organizations.

Salvatore Martini is a psychologist and a Jungian analyst. He is a member of the Italian Association of Analytical Psychology (AIPA) with which he collaborates in the context of its teaching activities, and of the International Association for Analytical Psychology (IAAP) for which he also supervises trainee analysts. Salvatore is a member of the Analytical Consultation Service of the AIPA and is active on the editorial board of the peer-reviewed journal *Psicobiettivo*. In addition, he teaches a course on analytical psychology organized by the Analytic Gestalt Institute (IGA). Salvatore collaborated for ten years in several mental health services, concentrating on therapeutic-rehabilitative 'integrated theatre' groups involving psychiatric patients and professional performers. This experience enhanced his understanding of the role of the body as an effective vehicle for expressing emotions and for unconscious communications, leading him to focus increasingly on the dynamics of embodied countertransference in his therapeutic practice. His paper 'Embodying analysis: The body and the therapeutic process' won the Fordham Prize in 2017. Salvatore lives and works in Rome, where he has a private practice.

David O'Driscoll works as a psychoanalytic psychotherapist for Hertfordshire Partnership University NHS Foundation Trust. This involves individual and group work with service users with an intellectual disability, as well as training and consultancy to staff teams. His background prior to working in the National Health Service (NHS) has been in social work with over 25 years of experience. He is conveyor for the intellectual disability section of the Association for Psychoanalytic Psychotherapy in the National Health Service (APP), founder member of the Institute of Disability and Psychotherapy (IPD) and is its current chair. He is also a member of the Social History of the Intellectual Disability Research Group based at The Open University. David is also a Visiting Research Fellow at the Centre for Intellectual Disability Research, Hertfordshire University.

Dr Valerie Sinason is the grandchild of refugees. A widely published poet, writer and psychoanalyst she is President of the Institute of Psychotherapy and Disability, Founder Director and now Patron of the Clinic for Dissociative Studies and on the Board of the International Society for the Study of Trauma and Dissociation (ISSTD) where she received a lifetime achievement award in 2016. *The Truth About Trauma and Dissociation: Everything You Didn't Want to Know and Were Afraid to Ask* (Confer 2020) won the Frank W Putnam award. *Trauma and Memory: the Science and the Silenced* was co-edited with Ashley Conway for Routledge (2021) and a first novel *The Orpheus Project* will be published by Aeon books in 2022.

Tom Wooldridge PsyD, ABPP, CEDS is Chair in the Department of Psychology at Golden Gate University as well as a psychoanalyst and board-certified, licensed psychologist. He has published numerous journal articles and book chapters on topics such as eating disorders, masculinity, technology and psychoanalytic treatment. Two of his articles were chosen as the 'Top 25' published in the past 25 years in the journal *Eating Disorders: The Journal of Treatment & Prevention*. His first book, *Understanding Anorexia Nervosa in Males*, was published by Routledge in 2016 and has been praised as 'groundbreaking' and a 'milestone publication in our field'. His second book, *Psychoanalytic Treatment of Eating Disorders: When Words Fail and Bodies Speak*, an edited volume in the Relational Perspectives Book Series, was published by Routledge in 2018, and has also been well reviewed. In addition, Dr. Wooldridge has been interviewed by numerous media publications including *Newsweek*, *Slate*, *WebMD* and others for his work. He is on the Scientific Advisory Council of the National Eating Disorders Association (NEDA), Faculty at the Psychoanalytic Institute of Northern California (PINC) and the Northern California Society for Psychoanalytic Psychology (NCSPP), an Assistant Clinical Professor at UCSF's Medical School, and has a private practice in Berkeley, CA.

Acknowledgements

I am extremely grateful to the newly relaunched Karnac Books for welcoming my proposal and for their interest in publishing this book. My heartfelt thanks to Ms. Christina Wipf Perry, Ms. Jane Ryan, Ms. Liz Wilson, Ms. Emily Wootton and to all members of the Publishing Team who have facilitated the production of this book.

I want to express my deepest thanks and appreciation to Brett Kahr, Valerie Sinason, David O'Driscoll, Gabrielle Brown, Salvatore Martini, Tom Wooldridge, William Cornell and Mark Linington for contributing with their chapters. Thank you for your enthusiasm and generosity in taking part to this project and for stimulating my own thinking and understanding of this very important and timely topic. My heartfelt thanks to Susie Orbach whose innovating thinking on the role of the body has much inspired me and who has honoured me by writing the book foreword.

I want to extend my gratitude to all the colleagues, teachers and supervisors who have motivated me to pursue my interest in this topic and who have provided me with the most helpful thoughts and suggestions.

Together with the other authors I would like to express my gratitude to all the patients whose clinical material forms a large part of the book's contents. In order to maintain confidentiality and protect their privacy, all clinical material has been disguised, unless permission was given.

Finally I want to thank my friends and family, whose love and support are always a source of joy and motivation.

Foreword

by Susie Orbach

Abject bodies

When it comes to bodies, psychotherapists, trained within psychoanalytic traditions, can struggle with the hierarchy of a theory which has, since the mid twentieth century, elevated mind, along with the complex intricacies of psychic operations, as primary or of primary interest. Body, has, sometimes inadvertently, sometimes purposefully, become, relegated to the symbolic register. It has been tasked with receiving the distressed and conflicted contents of mind as though body, the body, our bodies were a secondary or bit player to the principal drama of the mind.

Despite the early origins of psychoanalysis which stressed the importance of the body, this notion persists and is embedded in our practice. Outstanding researchers like Beebe (Beebe and Lachmann 2002) and Tronick (Tronick *et al.*, 1975). whose ground-breaking and beautiful work reading babies' faces for signs of connection and disconnection in early attachment, use the language of the body to describe the developments in infancy in almost entirely psychic terms. These developments are not only psychical, they are also developments in the appropriation of a bodily sense. Misattunements in body-to-body relating disturb not just a corporeal sense of the developing infant, they are taken into her or him as an insecure embodiment which is now destabilizing psyche. Analysts talk of holding environment as psychic space as though there were two minds at work. Today, the modern epidemic of disturbed eating and body image issues signals manifestations of body distress and insecure body development which need to be addressed and met in their own terms. Often we encounter these expressions of troubled bodies when we are visited by powerful body-to-body relationships in our consulting rooms.

In these revealing essays, we see the work of clinicians whose analysands have refused to leave the body in second place. We are plunged into accounts of a visceral engagement with the whole person – an engagement which can evoke difficult feelings in the therapist. As they tell of their encounters, we the reader are attuned to painful encounters which may make us retch, gasp and even revolt against what emerges from the page. And yet, this is so much our work. To hold, to be, to accept what can be so very difficult. We are there to receive the pain, the screeches and excretions; to find ways to make physical utterances – and their somatic impact on us – bearable and comprehensible.

The talking cure is profoundly physical; just as is our reading of these pages. Words enter us physically through what we hear in our ears, observe with our eyes, what we smell with our noses. We notice how breath and speech can be halting, consistent, staccato, screeching or, paradoxically, silent. Through registering how breath and speech are conveyed to us, we know that body is not simply a symbol. Sound, smell, vision are intensely corporeal.

Language itself, both the spoken word and the written word, are not mental constructs. That is too narrow an understanding of psyche-soma. Words are sound waves. Sign language is expressed via the body. The written word is physically transmitted through fingers. Language, in whatever manner it is delivered, is an expression of the psyche-soma struggle for subjectivity. It is not a lower order of subjectivity. Correspondingly – although not necessarily in a complimentary sense – the feelings that are aroused in us as we attend to the people we work with, are intensely physical and create the body-to-body relationship between us.

This body-to-body relationship is integral to the talking cure. Bodies emerge in the room when we are with people or on the phone and on Zoom. Our corporeality is not absent. We register feelings as part of beings. We are aroused physically and if we do not notice our bodies, if we are decidedly comfortable in our bodies working with a particular individual, that is in itself a diagnostic: the communication of what we might consider a Winnicottian good-enough body. If we are distressed when working with a person, the manner in which we experience our body countertransference will be idiosyncratic and unique to that individual. I am not talking of the therapist who falls asleep. That may be her symptom. I am talking of the experience of having an unexpected, enlivened body, a deadened body, a repulsed body, a false body, a misshapen experience. Powerful body countertransferences such as these are useful clues which can prompt us to the distressed embodiment of the people we work with. They can be seen as a glimpse into the disturbing experience of the person we are working with.

Mark Solms's epic work on consciousness (2021) resituates psychoanalysis on the ground of affects. And it very much helps us here. We could summarize this as: *We are because we feel. We feel therefore we are. We know because we feel.* We need no longer be mystified by how countertransference is conveyed to us. Solms sees countertransference as the registering of feelings in the therapist. And the essays in this fine collection stretch the envelope of feelings to include the abject, the uncomfortable, the disavowed, the screaming states of embodiment that we work with.

Here are the people we work with as they are rarely presented to a general psychotherapy audience. There is nothing tidy. This is messy, gruelling and yet deeply interesting and gratifying work. To encounter people who have so much distress around their corporeality and to describe them with such dignity as all the fine authors in this collection do is the best of what we have to offer. This is a humbling collection, a moving collection and a hopeful collection.

Use of terms

We appreciate that not everyone would use the same term for the person in psychotherapy, analysis or counselling. In this edited book the use of the term patient or client reflects the individual professional choice of each author. Both terms, in the context of this book, indicate a person that is receiving psychotherapeutic treatment either in private practice or in an institutional setting.

Introduction

by Raffaella Hilty

Every clinician will be well too familiar with what it means to experience the verbal expression of one's most vulnerable patients' distress, hatred and despair. But, what about those patients who cannot talk because they never developed the capacity to speak? Or those who are capable of talking but carry a complex range of unprocessed emotions that cannot be verbally expressed? These patients rely on another type of language to communicate their internal distress and, even though this is a topic not frequently discussed, many practitioners in the field of mental health have experienced working with people who communicate through the use of their bodies.

The body in its relation to the psyche has been a long-standing area of interest in psychotherapy. Starting from Freud and his early collaborators, up to contemporary thinkers of various analytic orientations, the topic of an embodied psyche has always attracted great attention and the hypothesis that somatic expressions can be found in place of verbal thoughts and fantasies has been central to psychoanalysis since its inception. In *Studies on Hysteria* (Breuer and Freud, 1895), Freud and his colleague Joseph Breuer used five clinical cases to demonstrate the psychogenic aetiology of the hysterical symptomology, positing that there was a symbolic relation between the physical symptom and the psychogenic causative factor. In their joint chapter 'Preliminary Communication' they write, 'It consists only in what might be called a "symbolic" relation between the precipitating cause and the pathological phenomenon – a relation such as healthy people form in dreams. For instance, a neuralgia may follow upon mental pain or vomiting upon feeling of moral disgust. We have studied patients who used to make the most copious use of this sort of symbolisation' (Breuer and Freud, 1895, p. 5). Among the various symptoms that constituted the diagnostic criteria of a hysterical neuroses they mention: 'neuralgia and anaesthesias of very various kinds,

... contractures and paralyses, ... chronic vomiting and anorexia, ... etc.' (Breuer and Freud, 1895, p. 4).

Freud's interest in emphasizing the relation between the body and the mind was likely rooted in his wish to provide psychoanalysis with a scientific biological foundation.[1] In his *Project for a Scientific Psychology* he writes, 'The intention is to furnish a psychology that shall be a natural science: that is, to represent psychical processes as quantitatively determinate states of specific material particles.' (Freud, 1895, p. 295). This intention is clearly expressed at least in three main areas of his work: his conceptualization of the instinctual drives, his explanation of the development of the ego and his theory of the aetiology of neuroses.

In *Three Essays on the Theory of Sexuality* Freud describes the instinctual drive as 'the psychical representative of an endosomatic, continuously flowing source of stimulation' (Freud, 1905a, p. 168). Later, in *Instincts and Their Vicissitudes* he refers to the instinct (*Trieb*) as 'a concept on the frontier between the mental and the somatic, as the psychical representative of the stimuli originating from within the organism and reaching the mind, as a measure of the demand made upon the mind for work in consequence of its connection with the body.' (Freud, 1915a, pp. 121–122) That same year in his paper 'The Unconscious' he writes, 'An instinct can never become an object of consciousness – only the idea (*Vorstellung*) that represents the instinct can.' (Freud, 1915b, p. 177). From these passages we can see that Freud considers the instinctual drive as the psychical representative of the stimuli originating from the body, as an emergent psychic function which, ultimately, remains unconscious because it is only the fantasy associated with it that comes into consciousness.

This view of the unconscious and of the instinctual drives as an area of contact between the mind and the body is also central to the thinking of Carl Gustav Jung, one of Freud's closest colleagues and 'crown prince' until their split in 1913. Jung refers to the instinctual drives as 'the psychoid' level of the unconscious or 'the psychoid nature of the archetype' (Jung, CW8, para. 419), a level of undifferentiated unity between psyche and soma. Like the instincts, the archetype remains in itself unknowable but it manifests endopsychically giving rise to archetypal images which are experienced as powerful affects. As a consequence, affects are the visible expression of the instincts and the bridge between the psyche and the soma. In *On the Nature of the Psyche* he writes, 'It seems to me probable that the real nature of the archetype is not capable of being made conscious, that it is transcendent, on which account I call it psychoid .... If so, the position of the archetype would be located beyond the psychic sphere, analogous to the position of physiological instinct, which is immediately rooted in the stuff of the organism and, with its psychoid nature, forms the bridge to matter in general' (Jung, CW 8, para. 417-420).

Another area of Freud's work in which the emphasis on the mind-body relationship is clearly coming through is his theory of the development of the ego where he postulates that somatic processes are the matrix for the development of the sense of self. In 'The Ego and the Id' he writes, 'the ego is first and foremost a bodily ego; it is not merely a surface entity, but is itself the projection of a surface' (Freud, 1923, p. 26), and in the footnote that first appeared in the English translation of 1927, he adds, 'the ego ultimately derives from bodily sensations chiefly from those springing from the surface of the body'. Similarly, his theory of the aetiology of neurosis, which roots all neuroses in the sexual history of the individual, is another area of his thinking that demonstrates the physiological foundation of the mind.

Freud was not the first to become interested in the psychogenic aetiology of hysterical neuroses. As Ellenberger writes, 'The circumstances that brought Freud to devise a new theory of neuroses belong both to the zeitgeist and to specific personal experiences.' (Ellenberger, 1970, p. 480). In the late 1800s it was Jean Martin Charcot who first identified the traumatogenic origin of hysteria and when Freud visited him in Paris at the Salpêtrière between 1885 and 1886 he was deeply impressed by him. Together with Charcot, another influential figure was Pierre Janet whose pioneering work on dissociation has paved the way for what is today known as dissociative disorders. The link between hysteria, trauma and dissociation is something that Freud and Breuer continued to explore. In 'Preliminary Communication' they write about 'the splitting of consciousness' which is 'present to a rudimentary degree in every hysteria, and that a tendency to such a dissociation, ... is the basic phenomenon of this neurosis.' (Breuer and Freud, 1895, p. 12). They observed that the memories of the traumatic experience, of which the hysterical symptoms were an expression, had become split off from the rest of consciousness. The treatment, at that time, consisted of helping the patient to abreact the 'strangulated affect' (Breuer and Freud, 1895, p. 17) through speech. When the split-off affects could become once again linked to consciousness there was a reduction of the symptomatology. Breuer's famous patient Bertha Pappenheim, known as Anna O., called this method 'the talking cure'.

Some of Freud's close collaborators, such as Sándor Ferenczi and Wilhelm Reich, made meaningful contributions to the study of the link between psychological trauma and somatic expressions. Ferenczi, for example, developed the concept of patho-neurosis and studied the non-verbal emotional expressions of people affected by trauma, as well as the reactions of people affected by organic diseases (Ferenczi, 1916–1917). Especially late in his career he engaged with the physical bodies of his patients, encouraging them to discharge their unprocessed traumatic experiences by entering altered states of mind. Reich, on the other hand, developed the concept of 'muscular/bodily armouring' or 'character armouring'. He theorized that, as the libido is ultimately a biological and bodily phenomenon so is the repression that opposes it, and he concluded that this mechanism of repression manifests in a pattern of muscular rigidity. This 'muscular armour' is a bodily pattern that expresses the emotional defence behind which lies the patient's trauma, so that there is a functional identity between a muscular rigidity and an emotional block. Both Ferenczi and Reich also introduced bodywork and stressed the critical importance of the therapeutic relationship to access and treat the embodied psychic blockages of their patients.

Another area in which the body in its relation to the psyche has been widely explored is the field of psychosomatic medicine. The Hungarian-American psychoanalyst and physician Franz Alexander, who was the director of the Chicago Institute of Psychoanalysis for almost 25 years, has often been referred to as the father of psychosomatic medicine due to his leading role in this field during the 1930s and until his death in 1964. Born in Budapest in 1881 he moved to Berlin in the 1920s where he became the first student at the Institute of Psychoanalysis and to officially qualify as a psychoanalyst. Overall, the psychosomatic approach acknowledges the contribution of emotions to the onset, course and recurrence of physical illness. As Alexander writes in the foreword to his book *Psychosomatic Medicine*, 'Every bodily process is directly or indirectly influenced by psychological stimuli because the whole organism constitutes a unit with all of its parts interconnected.' (Alexander, 1950, p. 12). Together with Freud, Ferenczi and Reich, Alexander developed the psychoanalytic understanding of the relation between the mind and the body, pushing the boundaries beyond the classic hysterical symptoms, where the dysfunction usually involves no physiological damage.[2]

From the above it is evident that Freud, his close collaborators and followers made great efforts to conceptualize an embodied psyche, where the body is seen as the matrix from which mental activity can emerge and where, on the other hand, psychological processes influence the physiological ones. Therefore, it is interesting that much of psychoanalytic thinking has often been criticized for its tendency to conceptualize the mind at the expenses of the body. A possible reason for this may be that free association soon became one of the fundamental rules of classic psychoanalytic technique, a method that emphasizes the importance of verbal language which may become implicitly seen as superior to non-verbal communication. In fact, whilst in *Studies on Hysteria* the focus is on the body that 'join[s] the conversation' (Breuer and Freud, 1895a, p. 296), and on the bodily symptoms that could be 'talked away' (p. 35) once verbalized and abreacted, by the time Freud published *Dora* (1905b) the focus seems to have already shifted to the patient's verbal narrative, and by 1913 the psychoanalytic method consisted in the analysis of the transference and of the resistance through free associations. As Jung put it in his paper 'The Theory of Psychoanalysis' published in 1913, at the time of *Studies on Hysteria* analysis was 'more or less closely concerned with the symptoms, that is to say, the symptoms were analyzed – the work of analysis began with the symptoms, a method abandoned today'. In addition, the 1940s and 1950s saw a turning away from the basic premises of Freud's drive theory, the bedrock of his argument for a biological foundation of the mind. Some of the main exponents of this psychoanalytic movement include Harry Stuck Sullivan, Clara Thompson, Karen Horney in the US and W. R. D. Fairbairn in the UK. What they all had in common was a belief that Freud's drive model had underemphasized the interpersonal context. Of course, Freud was aware of the importance of external relations but, to preserve the primacy of the drive, he had explained the role of the object in relation to its function of discharge of the impulse. The drive in this context is the determinant of an object relation. The new theoretical approach that emerged in the 1940s, instead, conceptualized object relatedness as the primary motivator of human behaviour and as the fundamental building block for the formation of the mind, a mind that develops in the context of a relationship. Specifically, Fairbairn criticized both Freud and Klein because, even though Freud's later work had placed more emphasis on the functioning of the ego and Klein had developed a theory of internal objects' relations, they both maintained that the aim of the impulse was pleasure seeking or discharge and that the object was just a means to an end. Fairbairn argued that the libido is inherently object-seeking and that the goal of the impulse is not pleasure or discharge but the relation to another.

During those years, on a parallel ground, the observational studies on animal behaviour led by the ethologist Konrad Lorenz, the psychologist Harry Harlow and the biologist Nikolaas Tinbergen, provided empirical evidence that the young of the species could become attached also to those adults who did not feed them, thus demonstrating that attachment behaviour is a primary psychobiological need, autonomous from oral satiation and sexual gratification. These discoveries deeply influenced John Bowlby and the development of attachment theory, where the infant is recognized as a human being predisposed to form relational bonds with others from the start. The subsequent studies of Mary Ainsworth (Ainsworth, Blehar, Waters and Wall, 1978) illuminated the importance of those early non-verbal interactions between the infant and the primary caregiver as the foundation for the development of the self, whereas Mary Main (1991) and Peter Fonagy (Fonagy, Steele and Steele, 1991), to mention a few, demonstrated how a reflective stance of the self towards experience develops from attachment security.

What I have tried to briefly outline above is that since Freud's alleged abandonment of trauma theory and the 1940s shift of emphasis from the intrapsychic to the interpersonal, psychoanalytic thinking focused on theories of the development of the mind and of the self in relation to another, paying less attention to the embodied dimension of the psyche. To quote one of the main exponents of contemporary relational psychoanalysis, Jessica Benjamin, 'The crucial area we uncover with intrapsychic theory is the unconscious; the crucial element we explore with inter-subjective theory is the representation of the self and other as distinct but interrelated beings.' (Benjamin, 1988. p. 20). More recently though, the influence of neuroscience on psychoanalytic theory (Damasio, 1994, 1999; Schore, 1994; Solms, 2015, 2021), new findings in infant research (Beebe and Lachmann, 2002) and a renewed interest in trauma theory (Van der Kolk, 2014; Levine, 2015), have brought back the attention to the body as the neurobiological matrix of the mind. The recognition of the reality of trauma and abuse in all its manifestations has prompted traumatologists and clinicians of various orientations to theorize once again about dissociation and somatization, whereas the influence of neuroscience on contemporary psychoanalytic thinking can be seen as a return to Freud's early mission to root psychological functioning in a biological framework, whilst emphasizing the interpersonal context in which the mind emerges.

Another very important area of influence that I believe is worth mentioning, is the work of contemporary clinicians such as Susie Orbach (1978, 1986, 2009), Gianna Williams (1997) and Jean Petrucelli (2015), in the context of eating disorders, Joyce McDougall (1989), in the context of somatic disorders and Alessandra Lemma (2010), in the context of body modification. These clinicians have made great contributions in bringing back the attention to the relationship between the mind and the body, a body that is often used or manipulated in perverse ways to maintain psychic survival, thus becoming the canvas on which one's story is told. Finally, I would like to mention the pioneering work of Valerie Sinason (1992) in the context of intellectual disability, that has illuminated the importance of bodily communications when working with people with no verbal speech but that can largely benefit from talking therapy.

All these influences, to mention a few, have contributed to rebalance the focus about the mind-body relationship, and contemporary psychoanalytic literature is filled with the efforts to conceptualize and treat the embodied dimension of the psyche. But, whilst relational psychoanalytic theory, mentalization theory, attachment theory and neuroscience all acknowledge the importance of the relationship between mind and body, that the mind develops from the body and that this takes place in the context of a relationship, I wonder if, in practice, once in the consulting room, this embodied dimension is something that is often still neglected today. How much do we truly pay attention to our patients' bodily symptoms or expressions and consider their possible psychogenic contribution and symbolic meaning? And how much do we pay attention to our own body and use it, like our unconscious, as an invaluable 'organ of information' (Jung, CW16, par. 163; Fordham, 1960, p. 247)? And when it comes to non-verbal individuals, do we automatically tend to exclude them from the possibility of talking treatment? Overall, I wonder if there is still an ongoing split in between what we say in theory and what we do in practice. This book wants to contribute to healing this split by providing a spectrum of clinical cases that demonstrate how one can navigate talking therapy when the patient conveys meaning through the use of the body instead of talking.

Primitive bodily communications can be thought of as embodied expressions of a disembodied psyche. What is expressed through the body are usually not neurotic conflicts but unmentalized affective experiences that, due to early attachment trauma or subsequent traumata, and at times in addition to an impediment of speech, have remained unsymbolized and unverbalized. Often these bodily expressions have been analogically described as *babylike* because, like in infancy, the emotional distress cannot be communicated with words and is expressed behaviourally and somatically. To quote Joyce McDougall, 'the infant's earliest psychic structures are built around nonverbal "signifiers" in which the body's functions and the erogenous zones play a predominant role. We are not surprised when a baby who is suddenly separated from its mother … reacts with gastric hyperfunctioning or colitis. When an adult constantly does the same thing in similar circumstances …, then we are tempted to conclude that we are dealing with an archaic form of mental functioning that does not use language.' (McDougall, 1989, p.10).

We acknowledge that the term *primitive* may convey a derogatory connotation. This is partly due to a long-standing psychoanalytic tradition that has framed bodily expressions as defensive, regressive and, either explicitly or implicitly, *inferior*. On the other hand we are also aware of the historical racist use of the word *primitive* in the context of a colonial Eurocentric tradition. However this book does not refer to bodily communications as *primitive* because we see them as *inferior* to verbal language, but simply because they point to the beginnings of psychological development, to primary ways of being and relating, as well as to enduring aspects of ourselves. Whilst on one side somatic manifestations are the result of a psychic defence organization to maintain psychic survival, on the other hand they are an intelligent and powerful way to communicate emotional distress. We want to highlight the important communicative aspect of these bodily expressions in the context of the therapeutic relationship, as well as their anticipatory role for the development of mentalized affects and, when possible, of their verbal expression.

The book explores the topic of primitive bodily communications in the context of intellectual disability, bodily neglect, somatic countertransference and eating disorders, and it is authored by contributors from various psychotherapeutic orientations, ranging across contemporary object relations, attachment, relational psychoanalysis and analytical psychology. Specifically, the chapters that refer to intellectual disability explore the additional challenges of working with non-verbal people and highlight the fact that, as much as the psyche affects the body so does the body affect the psyche, as the intellectual disability itself is traumatic.

Some of the chapters in this book include detailed descriptions of very ugly clinical material. Working with patients who communicated through spittle, defecation, urination, ejaculation and other bodily substances to convey unbearable affects, is something that confronts us, as clinicians and human beings, with the ugliest aspects of the work and of the human condition, those aspects that evoke in us horror, repulsion and disgust and that we wished we could avoid naming or dealing with.

In the opening chapter, Brett Kahr provides some historical perspective on the role of 'primitive bodily communications' in psychotherapy to introduce his work with a severely learning-disabled patient who spat compulsively, masturbated and urinated in the consulting room to communicate unthinkable, and unspeakable, emotional distress. Kahr masterfully describes a vast array of clinical material to demonstrate how he was able to engage with this highly tormented and traumatized person, eventually facilitating the remarkable improvements that he could observe after several years of psychotherapeutic treatment. In Chapter 2, Valerie Sinason provides an overview of her work with intellectual disability and extreme trauma. The clinical material shows how she compassionately engages with non-verbal patients who can communicate only through very extreme bodily behaviours, such as bleeding, head banging and defecating. This is followed by Chapter 3, where David O'Driscoll presents ways of working with people with an intellectual disability who self-harm. The first three chapters explore some of the most extreme forms of bodily communication when working with non-verbal patients, thus demonstrating how the 'talking cure' can work also with this population. Chapter 4, authored by Gabrielle Brown, explores the topic of bodily neglect. Brown discusses how individuals who neglect their bodily hygiene repeat scenarios of early abuse and neglect that are still dominating their internal psychic landscapes. She also explores ways of thinking about the meaning of smell and dirt from a socio-historical perspective and questions the long-standing socio-cultural attitudes that underpin a collective countertransferential resistance to understand this form of bodily communication. In Chapter 5, Raffaella Hilty discusses her clinical work with a patient who presented with a very unpleasant bodily odour, exploring the invasive and aversive aspect of this uncomfortable bodily symptom, together with its defensive and communicative function. Chapter 6, authored by Salvatore Martini, explores how embodied affects, resulting from a mind-body split rooted in early attachment trauma, are conveyed by the patient to the therapist in the form of somatic countertransference, which functions as an *organ of information* for the split-off complexes of the patient. The capacity of the therapist to enter a state of somatic *reverie* by dwelling in this third area as an intersubjective unconscious experience, allows the emergence of healing connections between the psychological event and the body. In this way, far from being seen only in their regressive and defensive function, the somatic symptoms, and our somatic countertransference, become harbingers of meaning. In Chapter 7, Tom Wooldridge explores bodily communications in the context of eating disorders, one of the most evident expressions of the use of the body to communicate unbearable psychic distress. Wooldridge revisits the notion of *the entropic body* (Wooldridge, 2018), a false body (Orbach, 1986, 2002, 2009; Goldberg, 2004) employed by patients with anorexia nervosa in an attempt to regulate catastrophic anxieties rooted in early childhood trauma which become concretized and expressed on their own bodies. In Chapter 8, William Cornell presents the clinical case of a young woman whose bodily symptoms included eating disorders and self-harm. Cornell explores how these somatic expressions narrated on the canvas of her adolescent body the struggle towards establishing a sense of adult personal and sexual identity, as well as anticipating psychic and interpersonal growth. The clinical material sensitively portrays the paramount importance of the therapeutic relationship in facilitating psychological change and interpersonal growth. In the final chapter, Mark Linington reflects on the possible Eurocentric colonial racist connotation implicit in the term 'primitive'. This points to a split of ego and id, rational and emotional, sophistication and uncivilization, and ultimately a split of the opposites which involves the disavowal of the 'other', the shadow, the 'not-me'. This split is central to the concept of trauma, which is a wound in the psyche. Linington refers to 'primitive bodily communications' as 'trauma-based communication', or communication of 'unfelt-feelings', and he presents two clinical cases, one of which portrays a person with dissociative identity disorder (DID). Here he describes how the dissociated and disembodied parts of the personality (personification of disavowed affects) used the body of the person's main identity as an object on which to express the unbearable affective experience of trauma. Linington discusses the importance of integrating those 'primitive' emotional states and ways of relating by bringing them in a more 'secure' relationship with the other coexisting aspects of oneself.

Notes

1. It is interesting to remember here that Freud's early work with his patients also involved physical engagement with the body (Freud and Breuer, 1895).
2. For example, in a hysterical paralysis the cause of the paralysis is psychogenic and the paralysed organ does not usually carry any physiological damage but is simply hysterically paralysed.

CHAPTER I

The spitting patient: speaking with sputum and free-associating with saliva

Brett Kahr

'Quod querulum spirat, quod acerbum Naevia tussit,
inque tuos mittit sputa subinde sinus,
iam te rem factam, Bithynice, credis habere?
Erras: blanditur Naevia, non moritur.'

['Because the old lady gasps for breath
And sprays saliva in your eye
And coughs as if she'd caught her death,
Do you suppose you're home and dry?
Miscalculation! Naevia's trying
To flirt, Bithynicus, not dying.']

Marcus Valerius Martialis [Martial], *Epigrammata* [*Epigrams*], XXVI

Communicating with bodily fluids

For those of us who work in the trenches of psychotherapy and psychoanalysis, we very much appreciate that the vast majority of our patients or clients or analysands will comport themselves with considerable dignity and maturity and, of course, with bodily *cleanliness*, during the course of a typical 50-minute session.

Although some of our patients will shout and curse, or rant and rave, or even bang their fists upon the arm of the chair or upon the surface of the couch, most of the men and women who consult with us will restrict their communications to ordinary verbalizations. Indeed, many speak with such fluidity and intelligence, whether reminiscing about their childhoods, pontificating about their dreams or revealing intimate details of their sexual lives, that I would describe the vast majority of psychoanalytical clients as truly linguistically *sophisticated*.

Needless to say, not all of our patients will free-associate in an unstoppable fashion. Some will experience moments of inhibition or silence. But, for the most part, our analysands speak to us with their mouths and their tongues, articulating word upon word in the privacy of our confidential consulting rooms.

During the 1880s, Dr Josef Breuer, the noted Viennese physician, worked with a young, hysterical woman, Fräulein Bertha Pappenheim, and he discovered, to his shock and delight, that by facilitating a number of ordinary conversations with this troubled patient, her neurotic symptoms gradually began to disappear. Fräulein Pappenheim came to describe her sessions with Breuer (1895, p. 23) as a 'Redecur', known, in English, as the 'talking cure' (quoted in Breuer, 1895, p. 23); and as a result of their frequent verbal interchanges, Fräulein Pappenheim experienced a veritable 'Kaminfegen' (Breuer, 1895, p. 23) or 'chimney sweeping' (quoted in Breuer, 1895, p. 23) of her rather cluttered mind. In 1895, Breuer published his remarkable case history of this hysterical individual, who has since become enshrined in the history of mental health as none other than the iconic 'Anna O'.

Breuer's experiences with Pappenheim exerted an immense impact upon the young Dr Sigmund Freud who, over the course of a lifetime, would elaborate upon Breuer's work and would develop the very foundations of the modern practice of psychotherapy, which we might describe, more accurately, as *talking* psychotherapy.

Nevertheless, in spite of the growing appreciation of the *talking* cure, our professional ancestors certainly came to recognize that not all of their well-educated, verbally competent patients would always free-associate in an unrestricted fashion. For instance, back in 1922, Dr Ernest Jones, one of the founders of the psychoanalytical movement in Great Britain, wrote to Professor Sigmund Freud about a female patient, Mrs Joan Riviere, who had undergone treatment with each of these men in turn and who would eventually become a noted psychoanalyst in her own right. However, in spite of this woman's intelligence, she often struggled, during her early days on the couch, to verbalize effectively, and Jones (1922, p. 454) recalled that, 'she was once dumb from Angst'. Fortunately, as a result of her treatment, Riviere eventually became quite able to 'talk fluently' (Jones, 1922, p. 454).

Subsequent practitioners discovered that even verbally inhibited patients would, in all likelihood, become better able to communicate in spoken language over time (Fliess, 1949; Khan, 1963; Winnicott, 1963). Indeed, some of our patients talk so rapidly, so extensively, and so profusely, that we, as practitioners, will often struggle to bring a 50-minute session to a conclusion. I suspect that we will all have had patients who have ended their psychoanalytical hour by pleading, 'Oh, just let me finish telling you about this dream that I had last night', or, 'Before I go, I must remember to mention that my partner and I had a huge row yesterday', or some similar sort of confession, desperate to extend the consultation by a few more seconds or minutes (or even longer).

As mental health practitioners, especially those of us who work either part-time or full-time in private practice with reasonably sane and sturdy men, women and children, we will encounter no shortage of sophisticated patients who engage brilliantly with the so-called 'talking cure'. Consequently, we readily devote ourselves to the facilitation of extremely warm and meaningful and rich conversations on an hourly basis with these individuals, often with great clinical success.

Not all of the people with whom we work, however, can be described as verbally sophisticated. Those of us who have toiled on the back wards of psychiatric hospitals and in the pits of old-fashioned mental health clinics know only too well that many of our patients do not communicate quite so readily in lucid tones. Some of our analysands will, in fact, relate to us in a very overtly *challenging* manner, which often evokes feelings of shock and, even, disgust.

As early as 1906, Dr Carl Gustav Jung (1906b, p. 7), the up-and-coming Swiss psychiatrist, wrote to Sigmund Freud, requesting assistance with a complex patient, namely, a twenty-year-old Russian female who had suffered from hysteria for at least six years, and who proved to be a 'difficult case'.[1] (In all likelihood, we suspect that this patient might, in fact, be identified as Fräulein Sabina Spielrein, a woman who ultimately became a psychoanalyst in her own right (e.g. Kerr, 1993; Richebächer, 2005; Launer, 2014.) Jung facilitated very detailed conversations with this young person and he soon discovered that, as a small child, she would often retain her faeces for weeks at a time and would then defaecate upon her own feet. Jung also reported that this girl had witnessed her father spanking her older brother, and he wondered whether she had developed a fantasy of excreting upon her father's hands, perhaps as an act of retaliation. Freud considered this case carefully and replied to Jung's letter, 'It is not unusual for babies to soil the hands of those who are carrying them.' (Freud, 1906b, p. 8)[2]

Over the next calendar year, as the collegial relationship between Jung and Freud became more professionally intimate, each man shared many other challenging vignettes about some very troubled individuals who would communicate in a rather primitive manner, not with words but, rather, with bodily substances. For instance, in the spring of 1907, Freud (1907) wrote to Jung about a male patient who screamed and who suffered from attacks of spitting, which the father of psychoanalysis regarded as a symbolic form of ejaculation. Likewise, this patient would run two of his fingers up and down a door, imitating coitus. This particular individual proved so impactful that Freud also wrote about this case to his German colleague, Dr Karl Abraham (1907) who had also consulted to this person. As Freud (1908b, p. 16) explained, 'His spitting is sperm-ejaculation.'[3]

These dramatic symptomatic manifestations continued to pepper the correspondence of the early psychoanalytical practitioners. Indeed, Jung (1907a) described the case of a young male catatonic patient, incarcerated at the Burghölzli asylum, outside Zürich in Switzerland, who would drink the contents of the chamber pot of another patient, consuming both urine and faeces. And not long thereafter, Jung (1907b) reported yet another catatonic individual – a female – who would smear her body with faeces. Furthermore, Dr Jung (1907c) wrote to Professor Freud about a woman who would vomit and, also, spit with great frequency.

Although these early psychoanalysts struggled to understand the meanings of such unusual and, often, revolting behaviours, they certainly did not dismiss the patients as unworthy of thought and theorization; hence, the correspondence between Freud and Jung provides much evidence of two pioneering clinicians who had attempted to unravel the secret meanings of these seemingly bizarre and insane forms of bodily behaviour. Thus, our ancestors within the psychoanalytical community certainly engaged from time to time with what Raffaella Hilty, the editor of this volume of essays, has encapsulated very helpfully as *primitive bodily communications*.

Freud had already written quite revealingly about the role of urination as a means of conveying powerful affects. In his landmark book on dreams, *Die Traumdeutung* (Freud, 1900a), better known in English as *The Interpretation of Dreams* (Freud, 1900b, 1900c), he described an episode from his own childhood in which, at the age of seven or eight years, he urinated in his parents' bedroom, prompting his father, Herr Jakob Freud, to lambast his son, 'The boy will come to nothing.' (quoted in Freud, 1900b, p. 216)[4] Alas, Jakob Freud had failed to recognize that his young son Sigismund's[5] act of urination might have represented a somatic communication of his sense of anger and, also, of his need for more parental care and attention. The young boy, however, regarded his father's comment as rather humiliating.

Throughout his own personal life, Freud would often communicate in bodily fashion by spitting regularly after smoking cigars. Indeed, he kept a brass spittoon in his consulting room (Kardiner, 1977; cf. Roazen, 1969, 1995) and would even spit upon a staircase from time to time (Freud, 1900a).

No doubt Freud's self-analysis and his own capacity to think about bodily fluids facilitated his work with subsequent patients, not least his noted obsessional analysand, Herr Ernst Lanzer, disguised as the 'Rattenmann' or 'Rat Man', who once fantasized about spitting in Freud's (1909b) face as an act of protest. Likewise, in the case report about the young phobic boy, Herbert Graf, immortalized as 'kleine Hans' or 'Little Hans', Freud (1909a) described the many ways in which this lad would spit as an expression of fear and anger.

Freud may or may not have appreciated how often references to spitting would penetrate his thoughts, even while corresponding out of hours with colleagues. For instance, when Sigmund Freud and his long-standing disciple Dr Otto Rank parted company due to a variety of theoretical and personal disagreements (e.g. Jones, 1957), Freud (1924) wrote to his loyal colleague, Dr Max Eitingon, about this matter, underscoring that his own daughter, Fräulein Anna Freud – herself a psychoanalyst at that point – had become deeply vexed by Rank's disloyalty. As Freud (1924) explained, 'Anna spits fire when the name Rank is mentioned.'[6]

Thus, Sigmund Freud would certainly have come to realize that young children and psychotic patients – who often lack the capacity to convey their anger and excitement in a fully verbal manner – will be more likely to communicate via actual spitting or urination or defaecation, whereas the more normal or more neurotic individuals, including his very own daughter, would spit with *words, rather than with saliva*. Although Freud never quite articulated the phrase 'primitive bodily communications' as such, he had, most assuredly, come to appreciate that those who lack the capacity to process complex emotions linguistically and intellectually will often resort to other means of expression.

Whereas Freud and Jung gradually recognized that speaking through bodily substances such as spittle might represent a secret means of expressing unbearable affects, the vast majority of psychiatric practitioners of the late nineteenth century and the early twentieth century dismissed spitting as a mere symptom of psychotic illness, which most regarded simply as a form of brain degenerationism. For instance, Professor Emil Kraepelin (1913), the veritable progenitor of biological psychiatry, considered spitting to be a core symptom of dementia praecox (the diagnostic precursor of schizophrenia), but offered no in-depth explanations of such behaviour in quite the way in which the pioneering progenitors of depth psychology had endeavoured to do.

Inspired by the work of Freud and Jung, many of the other founding figures in the history of psychoanalysis encountered patients who expressed themselves through bodily fluids rather than through spoken language. Thus, we have no shortage of case material about these patients who communicate bodily. For instance, Dr Montague David Eder (1924), one of the very first practitioners of Freudian psychoanalysis in Great Britain, produced a brief communication for *The International Journal of Psycho-Analysis*, in which he described a little girl who endured much separation from her father until the age of fifteen months, owing to his participation in the Great War. Upon the father's return from military service, this small child, who had suffered much paternal abandonment, would regularly defaecate into a chamber pot while perched in front of her father's feet. Although Eder did not elaborate upon this case in great detail, one can certainly hypothesize that, in view of the early ruptured attachment between the father and daughter, the act of defaecation might well represent both an attack by the little child as well as an attempt to establish some sort of link between these two individuals.

Other early practitioners followed suit and endeavoured to speak about this seemingly unspeakable topic. Dr Abraham Brill (1932), one of the pioneers of psychoanalysis in the United States of America, became one of the very first authors to write about the impact of bodily odours. Among the numerous clinical vignettes which Brill discussed in his paper, published in *The Psychoanalytic Quarterly*, he described the case of a psychotic patient who smeared faeces and who became so aroused by the smell of his own excreta that he would masturbate to orgasm in consequence. Likewise, Professor John Carl Flügel (1932, p. 59), a distinguished British practitioner, commented sagely upon 'bodily excretions', such as semen, urine, and faeces, as sources of potential symbolism.

Those psychoanalysts who, in particular, had trained previously in medicine, will have had no shortage of exposure to phthisis – namely, tuberculosis of the lungs – and, also, to haematemesis – the vomiting of blood. In consequence, it should hardly surprise us that Dr David Forsyth (1922, p. 7), one of Sigmund Freud's analysands, wrote about the ways in which a medical practitioner would facilitate a course of psychoanalysis: 'He will do best to train himself to regard every ebullition of emotion merely as a symptom, and just as he would never allow himself to be, let us say, angered by a persistent cough in phthisis or disgusted by haematemesis from a gastric ulcer, so these manifestations of feeling pass him by.'

Thus, by the start of the Second World War, the psychoanalytical community had encountered numerous cases of individuals who would communicate through bodily fluids. Those early practitioners certainly recognized that such enactments often, if not always, contain a great deal of unconscious meaning which must be both tolerated and, subsequently, explored in the consulting room.

In the post-war era, dynamically orientated mental health workers would continue to pontificate about such forms of primitive bodily expression in their clinical encounters and in their published case reports. The German-born psychoanalyst, Dr Frieda Fromm-Reichmann, who emigrated to the United States of America in the wake of Nazism, worked extensively with psychotic patients at the Chestnut Lodge sanatorium in Rockville, Maryland. In one of her essays, she underscored that the psychoanalyst must explore the hidden significance of the behaviour of ill patients: 'Your hair-pulling, spitting, and so on, does not convey any meaning to me. Maybe you can verbalize what you want to convey rather than act it out.' (Fromm-Reichmann, 1948, p. 268).

A highly experienced psychoanalyst, Fromm-Reichmann (1954) endured many encounters with patients who conveyed their emotions through bodily fluids, including one who urinated on the office chair. Another one of her psychotic patients, 'Mrs E', would defaecate on the floor and would also rip off her own clothing. Moreover, this person would spit, and claimed that, by doing so, kindly ghosts would materialize who would protect her from evil (Fromm-Reichmann, 1935). Strikingly, at least one of Fromm-Reichmann's colleagues at Chestnut Lodge, Dr Benjamin Weininger (1989), also had to navigate a patient who would spit at him. It seems that with institutionalized patients in particular, the use of saliva as both a weapon and also as a form of communication cannot be dismissed as a rarity by any means.

Likewise, Dr Alfred Schick (1948), an Austrian-born psychoanalytically orientated psychiatrist and psychotherapist who emigrated to New York City, New York, published an article about a case of psychogenic vomiting, in which a male patient would often discharge the contents of his intestines quite unexpectedly. Schick discovered that this adult man's vomiting would occur predominantly when he spent time at the home of his parents. Thus, the vomit represented a communication to the mother and father about feelings of hostility. In similar vein, the American-born psychoanalyst, Dr Charles Socarides (1969), treated a male patient who, as a boy, would spew up his food. Shockingly, this child's mother would force him to eat his own vomit as a punishment during his third and fourth years. Socarides expressed little surprise when he discovered that this former child vomiter had developed a sense of erotic arousal at the thought of choking his adult sexual partner by the throat, which Socarides conceptualized as a displacement of the patient's wish to have strangled his mother for having insisted that he consume his own childhood vomitus.

To the best of my knowledge, no one in the entire history of psychoanalysis or psychotherapy has written *in extenso* about the role of bodily substances and bodily fluids, per se, as forms of communication, in spite of the fact that various predecessors throughout the twentieth century have made fleeting references to this form of very primitive, archaic engagement. In the sections which follow, I shall now describe some of my own work with patients who have communicated with me through the use of bodily fluids, conveying traumatic distress in either a neurotic or a psychotic manner. I shall then present a very detailed case history of a woman whom I shall call 'Albertina', who would speak only through saliva.

Neurotic spitting and psychotic smearing

In an effort to provide a clearer clinical portrait of primitive bodily communications, let us consider three very brief clinical vignettes of two neurotic patients and of one psychotic patient, each of whom utilized bodily fluids of one sort or another as a means of conveying deep-seated psychological conflicts, and each of whom responded extremely well to classical, psychoanalytically orientated treatment.

The case of 'Gertrude'

Several years ago, I offered a course of psychotherapy to a very intelligent and highly accomplished woman called 'Gertrude'. Owing to her reasonably healthy childhood and her understandably considerable degree of mental health, Gertrude had no difficulty articulating her ordinary anxieties and fears through the traditional 'talking cure'.

In the course of our very first assessment session, I explained to Gertrude that should she wish to embark upon psychotherapy, it would be helpful for her to know about the structure of the clinical calendar in advance, and I thus explained to her that each year we would *not* meet for regular sessions during the month of August. Gertrude replied with great understanding, 'That won't be a problem. My family and I usually spend August overseas.' But, months later, as our very first summer break approached, Gertrude became increasingly infuriated at the thought that our psychoanalytical sessions would be interrupted by a 'holiday'. Indeed, in spite of her relative psychological sturdiness, she soon began to express much anger at the fear of missing out on one month of regular psychotherapy appointments, not least as she would have to spend a great deal of that time with her dying father.

In our penultimate session before the summer pause, Gertrude quipped that, in all likelihood, I had already made plans to luxuriate on a Caribbean island for the entire month of August, while she, by contrast, would have to devote herself to nursing duties, caring for her ill parent. At one point, she fumed, 'I am so envious of you, I could spit in your face.'

Because Gertrude already possessed a relatively healthy character structure, she could, therefore, readily transform her explosive emotions into straightforward words. Although Gertrude wished to spit in my face, she refrained from doing so in a concrete fashion; instead, she verbalized her aggressive emotions and her envious yearnings. As we analysed her fantasy of spitting on me, and as Gertrude spoke more fully, the anger diminished, and we then proceeded to embark upon many years of a rather successful course of psychotherapy (Kahr, 2021b).

The case of 'Millicent'

For a long time, I worked on a regular, twice-weekly basis with 'Millicent', a woman of 70 years of age, who impressed me with both her verbal literacy and her emotional intelligence. Sadly, Millicent had endured a very traumatic past. Not only had she survived the London Blitz during the Second World War, but she also had to navigate a painful separation from her parents who evacuated her to a home in the North of England. While in the care of a farmer and his wife, Millicent had to endure numerous episodes of child sexual abuse, as that older married man would often molest her late at night and would insert his penis into her mouth and ejaculate down her throat. As soon as the farmer left Millicent alone in the bedroom, she would then rush immediately to the bathroom in an attempt to expectorate the semen which he had lodged inside her oral cavity.

From the very outset of psychotherapy, Millicent would cry as she told me about her early experiences of sexual molestation, and she would even develop globus hystericus symptomatology in sessions and start to choke. Thereafter, she would reach for a box of tissues and then produce a staggering amount of phlegm which she would discharge into a clump of Kleenex. This anxiety attack recurred quite frequently during the first year of once-weekly psychotherapy, and Millicent seemed to have found the process of spitting into tissues rather cleansing, both physically and psychologically.

As we discussed those painful events from her childhood over the next few years, Millicent finally found a way to make some peace with the mental representation in her mind of the persecutory farmer, and, in due course, she no longer experienced such torment from the lifelong memories of the fellatio trauma. Eventually, Millicent stopped coughing up the semen-phlegm in sessions and, ultimately, had no further use for the tissues (Kahr, 2008; cf. Kahr, 2020b, 2021b).

The case of 'Steven'

Unlike Gertrude and Millicent, each of whom boasted tremendous capacity and intelligence and functionality, 'Steven', by contrast, though verbally fluent, had spent virtually the whole of his adult life on the back wards of a psychiatric hospital. I had the privilege of working with him psychotherapeutically over several years at a frequency of three sessions per week. Indeed, Steven had become my very first psychotherapy patient ever.

By the time I met Steven, he had already spent more than twenty years as a hospital in-patient, diagnosed as suffering from paranoid schizophrenia and, during more regressive periods, from catatonic schizophrenia as well. Indeed, he believed that the KGB planned to sodomize him with bayonets, and he also claimed that his private sexual thoughts would be broadcast aloud on both radio and television unless he committed acts of violence, such as punching the nursing staff or smashing the glass windows of the hospital. In view of this extremely persecutory ideation and the florid behaviour which ensued, it would be rather easy to overlook Steven's penchant for urinating in his trousers, and for arriving at sessions with large damp patches on his clothing. He would also blow his nose quite regularly without using a tissue or a handkerchief. Instead, he would pinch his nostrils and then exhale with great force, causing long strands of deep green mucus to emerge onto his upper lip. Steven would then rub the mucus into his beard and moustache and even onto the hairs of his chest.

Although Steven attended in-patient psychotherapy sessions several times each week, I did not encourage him to use the couch, in part, because of his lingering fear of being stabbed in the back, from behind, by both the Russian KGB, and also by the American Federal Bureau of Investigation. Instead, he and I sat in chairs, facing one another, thus affording me an all too clear view of Steven's urine-streaked clothing and his mucus-stained face. When I first watched Steven coating himself with these sticky bodily fluids, I had no psychological capacity to ponder the meaning of this symptom; rather, I nearly vomited from a sense of horror and disgust. Fortunately, I refrained from doing so. I suspect that many, if not all, young clinicians might have responded in a similar manner; indeed, whenever I described Steven's ritual in various teaching seminars in years hence, members of the audience would invariably develop a sickened expression from listening to these painful clinical stories, and, on one occasion, a colleague even began to hyperventilate, nearly vomiting in the process.

As our sessions progressed, Steven continued to squeeze the bridge of his nose, and would then blow hard, thus emitting large quantities of nasal mucus. I often wondered how Steven managed to produce such a markedly copious flow of that viscous, greenish substance. My patient proved such a stark contrast to the neurotic men and women with whom I worked in the outpatient clinic, many of whom would cry and blow their noses, but who always did so with the aid of a Kleenex. Steven seemed completely unabashed by his smearing behaviour, so much so that I found myself wondering whether he secretly *enjoyed* provoking a look of revulsion in the person observing his increasingly ritualized nose-blowing routine.

Over time, Steven continued to smear himself, but after I observed this behaviour on several occasions, I no longer felt nauseous or faint; instead, I took these bodily enactments in my stride as I began to metabolize the experience and ponder the reasons *why* Steven chose to smear at the precise moment that he did. Eventually, a number of possible meanings of this regressive activity began to emerge in my mind, and I started to verbalize my interpretations to the patient. Essentially, we explored two interrelated sets of potential explanations. First, I proposed to Steven that he may have covered himself with mucus in order to gauge my reaction, to see whether I could stomach him, in stark contrast to the father and mother who had arranged for his hospitalization so many decades earlier. Second, I suggested that, by smearing, he wanted me to know how dirty and uncared for he felt in the hospital, and that he must have worried whether I, too, would leave him to wallow in his mess. Steven smirked and winked at me, and then he replied, 'Shrewd, my good man, very shrewd. This place is a pigpen, and we are like pigs, wallowing in the muck.'

After several weeks of considering these interpretations, Steven finally abandoned his penchant for mucosal smearing in the consulting room and, to the best of my knowledge, this symptom did not recur after the termination of his course of psychotherapy (Kahr, 2012, 2021b).

Thus, having now learned about these very visceral cases – Gertrude, Millicent and Steven – one can readily come to appreciate that primitive bodily communications appear in a multitude of forms and that every psychological practitioner, regardless of one's professional background or theoretical orientation, must prepare himself or herself for such encounters over time.

Let us now explore the painful life of 'Albertina', a vigorous spitter with whom I worked psychotherapeutically over eight long years.

Spitting as a compulsive symptom: the case of 'Albertina'

The referral

I first encountered 'Albertina', a sixty-year-old profoundly mentally handicapped patient with challenging behaviour, during the early months of 1993. Apparently, this woman's much younger sister – the only other survivor of the family – had become quite distressed because Albertina had begun to assault several of the elderly, wheelchair-bound residents in the psychiatric facility in which she lived. The staff who attended to Albertina specialized in caring for the 'mentally handicapped' – those individuals whom we would now describe as 'intellectually disabled'; but, alas, in spite of their rich clinical experience, all of these professional men and women had begun to feel rather anxious and, also, extremely helpless, because they simply could not control Albertina's increasingly violent outbursts. For instance, from time to time, Albertina would purloin a metal frying pan from the kitchen, then sneak up behind some of the less mobile elderly patients and smash them on their heads, often inflicting quite serious bodily harm. Apparently, none of the staff seemed to understand quite why Albertina had begun to engage in such cruel behaviour; and nobody within Albertina's wider professional network of caregivers could ascertain what the precipitating cause or causes might be.

Albertina's destructiveness certainly served to compound the numerous forms of challenging behaviour and handicap that she had already presented to her family members and to the staff teams who worked with her around the clock. Not only did Albertina enact her violent feelings in such a destructive manner, but she proved to be a very difficult case in other respects as well, most particularly as a result of her compulsive spitting, and, also, her smearing of other bodily substances such as urine and vaginal discharges.

An essentially silent, mutistic person, Albertina would use her mouth in other ways. This sixty-year-old woman would expectorate extensively, upwards of a thousand times each day! The staff would complain that she would cover virtually every single item at her in-patient institution with strands of spittle. Albertina would also spit directly onto the faces of the staff members and the other handicapped residents, and she would spit on their clothing as well. She also spat extensively upon herself, rubbing puddles of saliva onto her hair and into her eardrums, as well as into her vagina and anus.

When not hitting or spitting, Albertina engaged in much smearing. As a younger, premenopausal woman, Albertina had a penchant for smudging her menstrual blood, in particular, on the floor and on the walls; she also smeared vaginal secretions and faeces, though not as often. The staff members never quite knew which form of bodily fluid would be used by this woman as an assaultive weapon. Although Albertina had spent more than 30 years as a psychiatric in-patient in a specialist residential mental handicap centre, the staff had become increasingly frustrated, and they threatened the sister, explaining that they would no longer continue to treat Albertina unless something could be done about her maddening and 'dirty' unmanageability. Naturally, numerous mental health professionals had attempted every possible variety of psychopharmacological and behavioural intervention over the years, including isolation and punishment; but, alas, none of those standard treatments seemed to have made any impact on the reduction of Albertina's destructive symptomatology.

To her great credit, Albertina's sister had begun to search the internet to educate herself more fully about different psychiatric and psychological treatment programmes for severely and profoundly mentally handicapped individuals who also presented with 'challenging behaviour', a euphemistic term then used quite frequently to describe such self-injurious and other-injurious activities as hitting, kicking, screaming, punching, head-banging and eye-poking, as well as spitting and smearing. Albertina had actually engaged in all of these forms of enactment. After months of researching the field of mental handicap, the sister discovered the work of Mrs Valerie Sinason (1992), a child psychotherapist at the Tavistock Clinic in London, who had only recently published a book on *Mental Handicap and the Human Condition: New Approaches from the Tavistock*, which documented the potential benefits of psychoanalytically orientated psychotherapeutic work with highly challenging disabled patients.

Fortunately, the sister promptly arranged for the Consultant Psychiatrist in charge of Albertina's care to refer this sixty-year-old person to the Tavistock Clinic's Mental Handicap Team, linked to the Tavistock Clinic Mental Handicap Workshop, to enquire whether a psychotherapist could be found for this very troubled woman. Soon thereafter, the members of the Mental Handicap Team convened to discuss potential new patients; and when Dr Sheila Bichard, an experienced educational psychologist, shared the referral during one of our meetings, all of my colleagues squirmed with great discomfort. None of the senior members of staff wished to undertake even a preliminary consultation with Albertina. But, as a young and naive practitioner, I offered to do so.

Immediately thereafter, several senior colleagues at the Tavistock Clinic urged me to arrange to receive an injection from my own general medical practitioner in order to inoculate myself against a potential hepatitis infection from this compulsive spitter. Another member of the team suggested that I should also purchase a great deal of plastic sheeting to cover the floor of my consulting room. And yet another colleague even recommended that I should acquire a spittoon.

I did, in fact, visit my personal physician to arrange for the hepatitis injection; but I felt instinctively that by covering my office with plastic sheeting or by installing a spittoon, such gestures might be experienced by the patient as rather unwelcoming and mistrustful in the extreme, and thus, I refrained from doing so. After careful consideration, I decided that I would meet with Albertina's sister in the first instance in order to discuss the possibility of offering psychotherapeutic work to this very troubled person. Needless to say, I felt somewhat anxious at the prospect of engaging with such a profoundly handicapped woman, burdened by so much overtly challenging behaviour, as I had never before encountered a disabled individual with this degree of damage. Indeed, in most of my previous treatments, I consulted with patients afflicted by mild mental handicap or moderate mental handicap issues. Nonetheless, I did feel partly fortified by the hepatitis injection, which seemed to provide me with some magical sense of protection against anything toxic which might emanate from Albertina.

In due course, the sister and I arranged a preliminary consultation, just a mere matter of weeks before the Christmas holiday in 1992. On the day in question, this woman rang the buzzer to my consulting room, albeit a few minutes late, and then climbed up the two flights of stairs to my psychotherapy office. As I opened the door, I observed Albertina's sister walking very briskly down the long corridor, puffing for breath, with numerous bulky and heavy shopping bags of every shape and size. Altogether, she carried six large parcels – three in her left hand and three in her right hand. As this woman neared the entrance to my consulting room, I introduced myself, and she did, likewise. The sister then ambled into the office and quickly relieved herself of these multiple, weighty bags, crammed full with brightly wrapped holiday gifts. She shook my hand firmly and exclaimed, 'Oh, what a relief to put down my Christmas shopping. I couldn't find a taxi anywhere and so I had to lug these bags halfway across town. I'm exhausted.' She then apologized for not having arrived precisely on time, explaining that she had great difficulty finding a parking space. Lumbered with six heavy parcels of shopping, the sister certainly could not have found a more dramatic and more heart-wrenching form of conveying the extent of her familial burden, having to care for such a disabled, handicapped elder sibling.

This sister's first set of communications seemed to have confused me. I wondered why this sibling chose to carry all of her parcels up two flights of stairs when, in fact, she could have locked these away in the boot of her car, not least as this woman had taken the trouble to tell me that she had arrived in her very own automobile. Although I do not often render psychoanalytical interpretations at the outset of an initial consultation with a family member, I did comment to the sister that perhaps by having entered the room with so many heavy bags and by having emphasized that she could not locate a taxicab, she wished me to know that Albertina proved to be such a very heavy weight and that she – the younger sister – might wish to find a 'car' or, indeed, a 'Kahr' (as in Brett Kahr), who could help her to bear the horror of this exhausting journey.

Albertina's sibling seemed to be hugely relieved and then responded, 'Yes, we are all rather hoping that you can do *something* with my sister. Anything would be helpful. *Anything* at all.'

After she seated herself in the consulting room chair, Albertina's sister then proceeded to speak to me about the family history. Apparently, in spite of having suffered from perinatal anoxia at the time of her birth, which may have resulted in some neurological damage, Albertina enjoyed, nevertheless, a relatively 'normal' childhood in a rural English setting, until the age of eight, when 'something' seems to have happened – possibly an experience of molestation by the gardener who worked on the family estate. The sister then spoke rather sheepishly and explained, 'Of course, Albertina is many years older than I am, so I wasn't born yet, but that's the rumour that went around.'

The sister then explained that, after this ostensible episode of sexual abuse, Albertina became increasingly withdrawn and sullen and stopped speaking in words; and, ultimately, she developed quite a 'bizarre' personality and would often bang her head on the walls of her bedroom. Some of her teachers would describe Albertina as 'slow'. By the time she reached puberty, Albertina had become a compulsive spitter and thus had to be removed from her local, state-funded school. Her family sent her instead to a special institution for the educationally 'subnormal', but, before long, Albertina caused so much disturbance that she ultimately required hospitalization in a psychiatric institution. She never again returned to the family home, not even for a single night.

As my conversation with the sister unfolded, I soon came to learn that, not long after Albertina had become institutionalized, the father, who struggled for many years with alcoholism, disappeared entirely and would never see either of his daughters again. The sister also revealed that their mother suffered from depression and, subsequently, from schizophrenia, and that, in due course, she, too, would spend many years in and out of psychiatric hospitals. It soon became quite clear that Albertina had endured much trauma, much abandonment, and much uncertainty, with little sense of security or safety. Her life history could readily be described as a litany of horrific experiences: born to a depressive, psychotic mother and an alcoholic, abandoning father; victimized by perinatal anoxia; molested, in all likelihood, in her latency years by a family employee; and displaced by a favoured sibling who – raised predominantly by a caring aunt and uncle – led a much more normal and much more fulfilling life. One can only speculate about the lack of protection that Albertina would have experienced in such a potentially chaotic family setting.

During our initial preparatory consultation, the sister seemed reluctant to attribute any of Albertina's symptoms to these aforementioned traumata. Instead, she argued that Albertina must simply have developed some sort of brain disease, in spite of the fact that, according to the medical records, none of the neurological investigations undertaken over several decades had revealed any positive, 'red-flag' findings. Naturally, while reflecting upon the sister's narrative, I soon began to wonder whether Albertina could well be an example of what Valerie Sinason (1986, p. 131) came to describe as '*secondary handicap*' (cf. Sinason, 1992), a concept which illuminates the ways in which many disabled patients had become handicapped *not*, primarily, as a result of organic deficits but, rather, in response to overwhelming psychological traumatization.

Before long, I came to appreciate the eagerness with which both the sister and the nursing team at the institution wished to surrender Albertina to my care, owing to the fact that all of these well-intentioned people had become extremely exhausted by this sixty-year-old woman who spent her days and nights spitting at her fellow patients and at all of the members of staff. The sister then emphasized that, at times, Albertina would become so distressed in her care facility that she would often scream in anguish, imitating 'the cries of a hyena'. Moreover, in addition to her unceasing compulsive spitting, Albertina continued to punch and kick both herself and the other residents not only with her hands but, also, with her feet.

The sister then explained to me that, more recently, her own husband – Albertina's brother-in-law – had threatened to leave her because she had to spend so much time visiting her elder sibling and, moreover, had to deal with all of the staff complaints. This well-intended but exhausted sister told me that if I *could* bear to offer some psychotherapy to Albertina – 'even just a few sessions' – this might actually help to save her own marriage as well. Needless to say, I became extremely concerned that the sister had communicated this seemingly unbearable level of distress. She then asked me whether I kept crayons and paints in my consulting room, explaining, 'My sister, Albertina, won't ever talk to you, but she does like to draw, so you might want to stock up on some more art supplies.'

As my meeting with this family member neared its conclusion, the sister stared at me in a forlorn manner and asked me directly, 'Do you think you can help Albertina?' I replied frankly that I would endeavour to do my very best and that it would be essential for me to meet with Albertina for an initial consultation, so that I could have an opportunity to assess her and, likewise, so that Albertina – a very frightened woman – could have an opportunity to assess *me*. I then enquired whether the sister had mentioned me to Albertina as yet, whereupon she explained that she had, indeed, done so and that, to her delight, Albertina did not throw a tantrum or engage in excessive spitting – her usual forms of resentment and protest. The sister and I then agreed that I would meet with Albertina the following week and that the patient would be escorted to my office by a member of her staff team. We also confirmed that if Albertina should wish to proceed with the process, she and I could, potentially, embark upon regular weekly psychotherapeutic sessions after the upcoming Christmas break.

As our meeting concluded, the sister turned to me with a hopeful expression on her face and sighed, 'It will be a relief to bring Albertina to a therapist. She really needs someone like you.'

The preliminary consultation

The following week, Albertina and her escort arrived exactly on time for our very first consultation. I must confess that no amount of prior work with handicapped, disabled individuals could possibly have prepared me for my initial sighting of Albertina. As she rounded the corner of the staircase and began to walk down the corridor towards my office, followed at close range by her escort, I caught a full glimpse of this very troubled person: a wizened and shrivelled – even emaciated – lady of some 60 years, who looked very much older, her head covered with long, frizzled, almost witch-like hair, which hung over her face in an out-of-control manner. Albertina could barely stand up straight, and as she ambled down the hallway with one foot turned outwards, and the other turned inwards, she kept banging up against the wall and almost fell over twice. The escort – obviously a very vigilant and attentive person – offered physical support. Albertina then teetered, as though quite drunk. Her spindly legs could barely support her large and gangly frame. I noticed that she wore a very untidy caftan, covered in dark, brown stains. In every respect, she looked exactly like the unkempt and neglected psychogeriatric patients with whom I had worked in hospital years previously, complete with very evident unplucked whiskers on her chin. In my case notes of this first consultation, back in 1993, I wrote, 'Albertina resembles a cross between the handicapped medieval monarch Richard III and the survivor of a Nazi concentration camp.'

At the threshold of my consulting room doorway, I introduced myself to Albertina and to the escort, and I then invited the new patient to enter. Albertina did not even look at me directly; instead, with bowed head, she staggered into my office and immediately fell down onto the floor, as though somebody had stabbed her. The escort leaned over and assisted the patient to her feet. I gestured to a chair, and the escort helped her into a comfortable seat. After this kindly woman had done so, she pointed to me, and then whispered to Albertina, 'That's Brett. He's going to have a chat with you. I'll be sitting outside while he talks to you. OK?' Albertina did not acknowledge the escort's words in any obvious way. This benevolent assistant then looked at me very sympathetically, as if to say, 'Good luck', and retired to the waiting room.

Tremulously, I sat down in my usual seat on the other side of the room, and I introduced myself once again: 'Hello, my name is Brett Kahr, and, as you know, your sister and, also, the staff members at your facility, thought it might be helpful if we could meet to talk about some of the difficulties that you have been experiencing.' Albertina buried her head abruptly into her lap, and she then began to rock in her chair. I waited patiently and silently, as I had no idea quite what I might say, partly overcome by the evident anxiety of working with such a distressed patient. Eventually, after watching Albertina rock back and forth for approximately two minutes, I spoke: 'It must be very strange for you to come here to this building to meet me for the ...' But, before I could even finish my sentence, Albertina leapt up from her chair, and, rather like a jaguar, with a newfound, sprightly dexterity, she lunged her body towards the other side of the consulting room and knelt down by the foot of the psychoanalytical couch.

Within seconds, Albertina returned to a standing position, and then, with great fury, she began to spit most dramatically, aiming strands of saliva at the wall of my consulting room. In retrospect, I can hardly remember how I felt at the time, as I had probably become somewhat numb from anxiety and confusion and shock. After aiming three or four mouthfuls of spittle at the wall, Albertina then expectorated onto the floor and, subsequently, she spat once or twice more onto her index finger, before ramming it into her right ear, making a very audible squishing noise. She would then lick her finger and expectorate several times more on the carpet. I simply could not speak at this point, because I found myself rendered quite silent as I watched this most extraordinary display of behaviour. She then covered the walls with some more fluids, and then spat, once again, on the consulting room floor.

After another moment or two, Albertina proceeded to spit into the palm of her hand, and then smeared the spittle onto the top of my desk. I felt nauseated, and, for a moment, I even wondered whether I would vomit – an undoubted countertransferential reaction of great magnitude. In retrospect, I can now better understand that Albertina wished to communicate to me how uncontained she felt and how she wished to violate the private spaces of other people, just as her own private spaces (i.e. bodily spaces) may have suffered invasion as a young, latency-aged girl.

Having now spat in dozens of places within the confines of my small office, Albertina then swept the great mass of hair out of her face, and, for the first time, she stared at me directly, as though investigating whether I might find her to be rather frightening or whether, in fact, I could bear to share the room with her. I looked at her with as much benign concern and curiosity as I could muster. She then fell down on the floor, once again, and soon crawled her way towards the small side table, located approximately two feet from my chair. In due course, she spied my appointment diary, located on the little table, and then, as she advanced towards this precious object (in which I would record the dates and times of all of my clinical consultations), I instinctively reached for the diary and quickly removed it from sight.

Undeterred, Albertina eventually teetered over to the other side of the room, and she dove underneath my desk and hid for several minutes. Ultimately, she poked her head out and then spat with even more vigour, in a projectile manner, onto my carpet yet again. She aimed her spits like missiles, and, within seconds, four or five messy puddles of saliva landed on the floor. This woman's capacity to produce such a copious stream of saliva quite amazed me. Once again, while still in hiding, she spat further onto her index finger, but this time, instead of sticking the finger into her ear, she jammed her digit under her caftan, and, to my utter surprise, she began to masturbate, touching not only her vagina but also her anus. At this point, I felt that I simply had to intervene, and I uttered, 'I can see how very frightening it must be for you to come here, and so you have been hiding under the desk to protect yourself, trying to find a way to bring yourself some bodily comfort when, in fact, this might be a rather scary new experience. And now you are demonstrating how much comfort and attention your body requires and that you need to take charge.'

Albertina seemed oblivious to my words, but, within a minute or so, she finally emerged from underneath the desk, and then she walked over to the doorway of my consulting room, and lifted up the entryphone, very visibly attached to the wall. She picked up the receiver, and, within a flash, she began churning her cheeks, manufacturing another puddle of spittle; and, with little hesitation, she then gobbed into the speaking part of the entryphone. I felt quite defeated by this point, and I began fantasizing about the cleaning fluids which the janitor of my building kept in a cupboard beneath the staircase. I knew only too well that I would have to invest a great deal of time and effort in order to remove all of the spittle from the carpet and from the walls.

Undeterred, Albertina resumed spitting into the receiver of the telephone. Exhausted and overwhelmed by this unprecedented consulting room behaviour, I suddenly realized that I might, at last, have something more useful to say. My psychoanalytical thinking process returned to me, and, thus, I offered the following formulation: 'As I have said, I know that you must be scared. You do not know whether I am a safe person or whether I will harm you in some way. And you are here in an unfamiliar room that you have never visited before, and you might be wondering why you have been brought here. I think that you are covering the entire room with spit to make it your own, so that it becomes a safe place. And I think that by spitting into the telephone, as you are doing now, you are trying to find a way to talk to me. I know that it is difficult for you to speak in words, as I am doing, so you are using your spit as a way of communicating with me.'

To my huge relief, this verbal intervention did seem to have an impact on the sixty-year-old Albertina. Upon absorbing my words, she dropped the entryphone immediately and left it dangling; she then ambled her way to the middle of the consulting room and slumped down on the floor in a heap, and then she began to cry. The patient did not sob in an audible way; instead, a trickle of tears streamed silently down her cheeks, and she looked very sad indeed. Suddenly, the emotional atmosphere altered quite considerably, as I (and, perhaps, Albertina as well) experienced considerable hope that the madness and the acting-out could be contained, and that something might be understood. She did not reply to me in words, but, as she sobbed, I spoke to her: 'I can see how very unhappy you are, and I think that there is a part of you that wants help. But you are also wondering whether I will be able to help you, and whether you can trust me to help you, or whether you have been sent here by your sister and by the staff members as some kind of punishment.' Albertina looked up at my face and she continued to cry.

In this respect, Albertina certainly demonstrated that, in spite of any neurological or cognitive consequences of the perinatal anoxia, she possessed, nevertheless, the ability to understand my words and, also, the developmental capacity to move from a more tortured, persecuted state of paranoid-schizoid functioning, wherein she experienced the world as a dangerous place, to one of more depressive functioning, in which she could recognize the true sadness of her existence (Klein, 1946; cf. Klein, 1935). Many clinicians would regard the presence of such depressive potentialities – epitomized by her tears – as a great psychological achievement (cf. Hinshelwood, 1994; Anderson, 1997).

Eventually, Albertina dried her eyes and then extended her hand and spat gently onto her palm. Within a matter of seconds, she proceeded to rub some saliva into her scraggly headful of greying hair, twirling some of the strands around and around in a repetitive and compulsive manner. I became aware that this particular act of spitting seemed rather different from her earlier, more aggressive expectoration activities; indeed, I wondered whether Albertina used projectile spitting not only as an expression of hostility but, also, as an attempt to ward off fear and, additionally, as a form of comfort, and as a means of containing her extensive anxieties. It then occurred to me that speaking with saliva might well have become Albertina's primary *language*. I therefore came to appreciate that, in order to work with this very troubled person, I would have to learn how to decipher her very unique language, which I came to refer to as 'spittingese'.

As this initial psychotherapeutic interview drew to a close, Albertina and I looked at one another very plaintively, neither of us entirely certain what, precisely, had unfolded during our very first encounter. In a soft voice, I explained that we would have to conclude our meeting in a short while, but that we needed to decide whether she might wish to visit me every week, so that, together, we could do our best to think about her situation. Extraordinarily, Albertina did not look up at me; instead, she surprised me by removing her shoes and then her socks. I rendered yet another interpretative comment, 'I have just mentioned that we shall have to finish soon, and you have just taken off your shoes and socks. Perhaps you are showing me the part of you that *does* want to stay here and not leave me.' Albertina then started to rock back and forth once again, exactly as she had done earlier in the session.

Quietly, I explained that it would be important for her to put her shoes and socks back on, and that she could certainly spend some time during the upcoming days reflecting on our meeting, and that, next week, we would decide jointly whether it might be helpful for her to come to see me on a regular basis. Albertina then stood up, grabbed her shoes and socks, and walked towards me in a purposeful way, handing me her footwear, just like a small child who wishes for a parent to help him or her to dress. I replied that, as I had already seen her take off her shoes and socks, I knew that she could probably put them back on by herself, underscoring once again that perhaps she wished to communicate that she does want my assistance.

Silently, Albertina sat back down on the floor and, in a slow, laborious and frustrating manner, she spent approximately three or four minutes more putting her socks and shoes back on her feet. I waited patiently and then stood up from my consulting room chair. I opened the door and I nodded to the calm and containing escort, seated outside in the waiting room area. This benign-looking colleague then walked into the office, saw Albertina seated on the floor, and asked her in a sympathetic way, 'Well, how did it go?' Of course, Albertina did not reply in words, but she did stand up on her feet, and thus prepared herself to leave the room. I then addressed the escort: 'I have explained to Albertina that it will be helpful for her to think about this first meeting during the week. And then, next week, we can meet again at this same time and decide whether she might wish to see me on a more regular basis.' The escort nodded in affirmation, and she and Albertina then began to depart. The escort turned to Albertina and encouraged her, 'Say goodbye to Brett.' Albertina looked at me in silence, but she did make some eye contact. I then said, 'Goodbye. I shall look forward to seeing you next week.'

As soon as I closed the door, I breathed an audible sigh of relief and attempted to compose myself. Some minutes after Albertina and the escort had left the building, I then went in search of the cleaning equipment, and, after having discovered a pile of brushes and cloths and sprays, I began to scrub the carpets and walls of my room with great vigour, trying to remove the very evident spittle stains. I estimated that Albertina must have spat more than 200 times during our first 50-minute meeting. I wondered seriously whether I would be able to assist her in any way and whether, in fact, I really ought to engage with such a highly disturbed patient.

The following week, Albertina and the escort returned at the appropriate time; and although this most unique patient spat continuously throughout the session, I later estimated that, during our second meeting, she might have spat only 100 times, or thereabouts, as opposed to the more than 200 episodes of spitting which had occurred during the first session, thus suggesting to me that the engagement with a psychotherapeutic structure might well help to contain some of her more unprocessed and undigested affects (cf. Bion, 1962a, 1962b). As the second consultation session unfolded, I enquired of Albertina whether she had any thoughts about coming to see me on a regular basis. She responded by staring at the wall and by rocking, but she certainly did not reply in any overt, verbal manner. However, after two or three minutes, she picked herself up, walked over to the entryphone, and then spat into the receiver once again, just as she had done during her first consultation the previous week. I interpreted that although she harboured mixed feelings – even angry feelings – about her sister and her staff team for having recommended that she should meet me, she also wished to convey the part of her which does, indeed, crave help and assistance from someone who can respond to her 'telephone calls'.

I explained to Albertina that I would be able to meet with her for a regular weekly session at this exact time, beginning in the first week of January, 1993. I then described all the practical arrangements to her, such as the typical clinical calendar which would incorporate a pause in the work at Easter, and during the month of August, and, also, at Christmas. Albertina seemed to nod her head, albeit in a very ginger manner.

We then launched upon our work ... with much trepidation and uncertainty.

I hasten to add that, in order to help me deal with this very complicated patient, I arranged to receive clinical supervision for my work from a very esteemed psychoanalyst, who had practised for many years with both adult patients and child patients. I suspected that a psychoanalyst who had treated people of every age could be of great value in helping me to understand my clinical interactions with Albertina, a sixty-year-old woman in the chronological sense, but a baby in the psychological sense, who spent much of her time spitting up the symbolic maternal milk in the form of saliva. Not knowing whether I had actually undertaken the treatment of an older woman or of a small infant who could not keep her bodily fluids inside of her, I felt very contained by the anticipated support from both my clinically esteemed supervisor and from my colleagues at the Tavistock Clinic Mental Handicap Team and, also, those in the

Tavistock Clinic Mental Handicap Workshop, with whom I met weekly in a special discussion group, created by Valerie Sinason and run along psychoanalytical lines, in which an experienced community of disability clinicians would discuss complex cases of this variety.

In reviewing my first two meetings with Albertina, I did come to appreciate that although this patient had presented herself in a very wild and crazed fashion, she also demonstrated most clearly that she possessed the capacity to become more contained, particularly after I had offered a reflective or interpretative comment, thus illustrating very vividly what the pioneering psychoanalyst, Mrs Melanie Klein (1932), had highlighted many decades previously, about the potential for a verbal interpretation from the clinician to reduce the patient's level of anxiety. With this knowledge in the forefront of my mind, I felt much more ready to proceed with our weekly psychotherapeutic sessions.

The treatment

Happily, and quite unexpectedly, Albertina really did begin to engage with the process. Her exceptionally reliable and professional escort drove her to my consulting room every single week, without fail, and never, ever arrived even one minute late. Although Albertina did not, or could not, speak in words, as most normal-neurotic patients would do, she did communicate in a wide variety of ways, whether through spitting or through other forms of behaviour. In fact, she became so very immersed in our appointments that she and I continued to meet on a weekly basis for fully *eight years*. Naturally, one cannot readily summarize over 300 sessions of psychological encounters in such a brief context; therefore, I shall focus, instead, on three key themes and images and motifs which emerged over time and which, I hope, will provide some flavour of the interactions between the two of us.

1. Spitting

If we concentrate solely on the act of spitting – arguably the most noticeable, persistent, and disturbing of Albertina's presenting symptoms – I gradually became aware of some very marked changes over the course of nearly a decade of ongoing psychotherapeutic work. As I have already indicated, throughout the very first assessment session, Albertina spat on more than 200 occasions, covering not only the walls and carpets in the consulting room with spittle but, moreover, her own body. Strikingly, across our long working relationship, Albertina never expectorated on me, partly due to fear but, also, perhaps, as a means of preserving me as a good object in her internal world. During the second assessment session, she spat roughly half that amount, maybe 100 times or thereabouts. To have observed such a huge reduction in this symptom – 200 spits in the first meeting and 100 spits in the second appointment – provided me with some hope that this very troubling and endangering symptom could be contained, minimized and, possibly, even cured.

To my great relief, and to the immense delight of Albertina's family and caretakers, the sheer quantity of spitting continued to decrease dramatically, both in the psychotherapy sessions and, also, in her psychiatric institution. Indeed, by speaking about the spitting during our consultations and by offering psychoanalytical interpretations of the potential meaning of different acts of spittle, I believe that I might have created a growing atmosphere of reliability and safety which could have contributed to the diminution of her vexing symptomatology.

During the first year of treatment, I often felt that I simply had little option but to tolerate the spitting, as it occurred so regularly throughout our work, perhaps 50 or 60 times per session across the early months – roughly one episode of spitting each minute. Fortunately, I maintained a sense of hope by constantly recalling that the spitting served not only as an act of *hostility* but, also, as a form of *communication* for this mutistic patient, and that it seemed to be linked to anxiety, and could, thus, be reduced through the formulation of a classical psychoanalytical interpretation. Nonetheless, throughout the early phase of treatment, I often had to combat waves of nausea as I watched Albertina expectorate on her fingers, on her hands, and on all sorts of objects in my office, including my much-cherished bookcases on at least two occasions. Invariably, she would manufacture the spittle in her mouth, gob it onto her finger, and then penetrate her ear with her moistened digit, simulating the thrusting movements of a penile object. Naturally, I did remember only too clearly my initial meeting with Albertina's sister who spoke about the sexual trauma which the patient might have endured in her latency years, decades previously. The image of the saliva-drenched finger jabbing in and out of her aural cavity certainly conjured up images of abusive penetrative intercourse.

Needless to say, I found myself quite preoccupied with the possibility that her spitting may have come to represent a symbolic re-enactment of an earlier sexual molestation, but I also sensed that these acts of spitting might have other meanings as well; therefore, I struggled and thought carefully before I made any interpretation which might crudely reduce all of the spitting to merely one simple explanation. As the work unfolded, I gradually came to realize that the spitting occurred at different moments, and at variable intensities, throughout the course of the psychotherapy session, and I came to appreciate that one of my principal, ongoing tasks would consist of the continuous close monitoring and fine-tracking of these spitting episodes, in an attempt to ascertain the particular significance of a certain bout of expectoration.

For instance, whenever Albertina would salivate on her finger, and then penetrate her eardrum – sometimes drawing blood in the process by having bruised the skin on the outer ear – I often found myself commenting: 'You are ramming your finger into your ear in a very hard way, and it looks as though you are hurting yourself very painfully. I wonder whether you are trying to show me that perhaps somebody else had once put something hard and wet and hurting into a part of your body.' As with many of the interpretations that I articulated with this predominantly silent psychotherapy patient, I often had to repeat the same words over and over again, across the long months and years of treatment. When I first began to talk to her about the meaning of inserting her saliva-streaked finger into her ear, Albertina became wild, and she would run to the other side of the room, or she would rush to the couch, grab the pillow, and stick it over her head so that she could not hear me speaking; occasionally, she would ram her finger into her ear even more deeply and more frantically in response, in order to ensure that she could not consider my hypotheses at all. Fortunately, as the treatment progressed, Albertina eventually ceased attacking her body in this way and, after three years of sessions, would no longer engage in any finger-thrusting behaviour; instead, the patient would look at me with her sullen, droopy, depressed face, acknowledging with the poignancy of her eyes the full reality of what I had interpreted about the potential of an early sexual attack by an older man.

Sometimes, Albertina deployed her spittle in other ways, and for other purposes. For example, she often used saliva as a possible means of communicating some experience of bodily invasion and, also, as a form of attack. At the end of each appointment, I would announce the time, and would begin to walk across the room in order to open up the door, so that Albertina could thus be reunited with her escort, who always sat quietly in the nearby waiting room. At precisely those moments of transition, Albertina's spitting would often become exacerbated, and, as the sessions drew to a close, she would start to spit with savage fury – rather like a machine gun – producing one glob of spittle after another, as a means of expressing her fury.

Throughout the treatment, I detected at least one other possible meaning of Albertina's spitting, namely, that such behaviour might serve as a vehicle for testing whether I could actually tolerate her physical presence. From time to time, Albertina would drench her finger in spittle and would then approach the chair in which I always sat. With a look of devilishness on her face, she would smile through her mass of tangled hair and would then touch the arm of my seat gingerly with her wet, saliva-soaked finger. After she had done so, she would run rapidly to the other side of the room and would hide behind my desk. In response, I would often interpret: 'You really want to know what will happen if you spit on my chair. Perhaps you have run away because you are worried that I might punish you or hurt you in some way. Perhaps you are relieved that I have not become angry in the way that many people often do when you spit on their chairs.' Of course, from time to time, I did find myself becoming very internally cross with her for spitting in my room, or for streaking the arm of my chair with saliva; but I did manage to recognize that Albertina wished to see exactly what I might do when confronted with her saliva in this way and whether I could bear it. After I made my interpretation, Albertina would often smile cunningly and would then reappear from behind the desk before returning to the centre of the room, reassured that I had not retaliated at all.

Those early spittle explosions across the first years of treatment could best be understood as expressions of both aggression and desperation and, perhaps, as re-enactments of early traumata. Strikingly and, perhaps, unsurprisingly, Albertina's primitive bodily communications provoked a sense of nausea in me during the early stages, as I had never before witnessed another patient spitting approximately 200 times in the course of 50 minutes. One might describe such a private reaction as a form of somatic countertransference. In her iconic studies of nausea as a countertransferential expression, Valerie Sinason (1988, 1992) – the leading progenitor of disability psychotherapy in the United Kingdom – theorized that nausea will often arise as an unconscious reaction to an unprocessed case of child sexual abuse.

Inspired by Sinason's work on the role of somatic countertransference as an indication of early traumata, I thus began to name the unnameable (cf. Sinason, 1991), and would wonder aloud with Albertina whether she might have wished to communicate her own sense of bodily unsafety by making others feel soiled. In doing so, my nausea gradually dissipated, as did any further manifestations of Albertina's very destructive episodes of painful ear-poking behaviour. Thankfully, as our work progressed across the years, Albertina felt increasingly safe with me in the privacy of the consulting room and, consequently, she soon began to internalize an experience of being physically unharmed and treated with bodily respect.

Hints about the possibility, indeed probability, of early sexual abuse would emerge continuously throughout the treatment. On one occasion, Albertina entered the consulting room and then lay down on the couch, whereupon she proceeded to seize the pillow and thrust it over her face, enacting some sort of smothering ritual. She then started to buck her hips up and down in a most violent fashion. I could not help but imagine that she wanted me to see that somebody had taken a pillow and silenced her, and had then, perhaps, penetrated her body. Whatever difficulties Albertina had endured with a depressive and, even, schizophrenic mother and with an alcoholic father, I felt confident that she wished me to know about other forms of intrusion, invasion, and penetration as well, inflicted, in all likelihood, by the family gardener.

In a lecture to colleagues at the Tavistock Clinic Mental Handicap Workshop, I outlined a four-stage process of digesting the powerful emotions and symptoms revealed by extremely disabled patients such as Albertina who evacuate bodily fluids in sessions (Kahr, 1995; cf. Kahr, 1996, 1997, 2020a, 2021b). I suggested that when first presented with the full aggressivity and traumaticity of the fluid – in this case saliva – one becomes attacked oneself and will thus struggle to think in a deep and symbolic manner. I identified this as the *stage of stupefaction*. Eventually, through supervision, through discussion with colleagues, and by processing the meaning of these powerful symptoms and affects, the clinician will begin to develop a growing capacity for *toleration*; and the strong, often overwhelming, countertransferential reactions, such as nausea, will gradually diminish, thus permitting one to bear being in the room with the patient more fully. Eventually, the third stage can be reached, namely, that of *interpretation*, wherein the psychotherapist attempts to translate the unconscious meaning or meanings of the patient's behaviour, resulting, ultimately, in the fourth stage, which one might describe as a *resolution*, or working-through, of the ongoing primitive symptoms.

The unravelling of Albertina's spitting compulsion adhered to these four stages precisely. Beginning with 200 spittles or more throughout our first consultation, the rate of expectoration decreased steadily across the course of treatment. After one year of psychotherapy, the patient managed to contain herself sufficiently so that on average she spat only 20 to 30 times per session. I would estimate that after two years of our psychotherapeutic work, the rate of the patient's spitting decreased to some 10 or 15 spits per session; and, over time, this number continued to diminish even more so. Thankfully, after approximately six years of regular weekly psychotherapy, Albertina would spit only once per session. Not long thereafter, during the latter part of the sixth year of treatment, the spitting stopped *completely*, much to the relief of all the nurses and care workers and mental health professionals who had to tend to Albertina on a daily basis.

It might be of some interest to learn that, during one of our sessions in the seventh year of consultations, Albertina had not spat at all. As our 50-minute hour neared its conclusion, I sneezed, quite audibly, and quite uncharacteristically, for the very first time. I do not usually sneeze in the course of psychotherapeutic work, and this reaction surprised me. Albertina responded very strongly to my sneeze and stared at me with a look of consternation, and then started to slap herself around the face, something that she would do rather frequently during the first year of treatment but had not done for quite some time. The patient then stood up from the couch, upon which she had perched herself, and then hawked a great big globule of saliva onto the carpet, once again, something that she had not done in such an obvious way for more than a year. In response to this regressive behaviour, I ventured an interpretation: 'I think you felt very hurt and angry when you heard me sneeze a moment ago. I think you felt that I might not have been thinking about you or paying attention to you in that moment, but rather, that I had been concentrating on my own sneezing. I think that you started to hit yourself because you really wanted to hit *me*, and I suspect that you may have spat upon the floor of the office in order to show me the extent of your anger.'

I do not know what sense – if any – Albertina might have made of my interpretation, but I did come to learn that one must be extremely sensitive and must endeavour to understand why this patient would spit at such a precise and particular moment within the course of a session. Indeed, I endeavoured to draw upon the experience of having studied infant observation during my training (e.g. Bick, 1964; Harris, 1987; Rustin, 1989; Miller, 1999), which helped me to understand more fully the meaning of a small piece of material within a particular context. I have a strong sense that Albertina came to appreciate this fine tracking and monitoring approach, and that this very detailed vigilance assisted me very much in my formulation of more accurate verbal interpretations which helped to alleviate her anxiety and her behavioural enactments through primitive communications (e.g. Klein, 1932; cf. Rosenfeld, 1987).

2. Crayons and drawings

At the outset of treatment, Albertina communicated through spitting and through silence, and she produced virtually no audible sounds at all. Occasionally, the patient would wail and scream, particularly at the end of sessions, but, on the whole, she remained electively mutistic. During the preliminary meeting with Albertina's sister, she had mentioned to me that her elder sibling enjoyed drawing. She also informed me that, in all likelihood, Albertina would not speak to me in words, even though, as a child, she had acquired some language and she certainly understood human speech. Although I do not ordinarily work with drawings or art materials, as I prioritize the more classical psychoanalytical procedure of facilitating deep conversation, I did place a small pad of paper and a slender box of crayons within Albertina's sight, perched unobtrusively on a little nearby table.

Albertina avoided the crayons during the very first month of treatment, but, in the fifth session of psychotherapy, she became intrigued and, on one occasion, she lifted up the cardboard box with seeming interest. Albertina then fiercely ripped open the container of crayons, and she threw the cardboard wrapping aside, thus permitting all the crayons to scatter across the floor. She then grabbed the pad of paper and tore off the cardboard backing and flung it across the room as far as she could with strong arm gestures. Eventually, Albertina picked up a black crayon from the floor and brusquely broke off the pointed tip, which she flung towards the rubbish bin. Albertina then sat down in the middle of the floor, clutching this tipless, castrated black crayon, and she proceeded to draw a single stroke on a page of the mangled paper.

Deeply ensconced in this new activity, Albertina drew a thin line which ran from the upper left-hand corner to the lower right-hand corner of the page and, for the next ten minutes or so, she continued to trace the line backwards and forwards in a repetitive fashion. I sat silently and observed her attempted artwork. I must confess that I found myself becoming slightly sleepy in the process. After all of those spirited and energetic attacks on the crayon box, and on the cover of the writing pad, and, also, on the tips of the crayons, I had a sense that Albertina had already discharged quite a large amount of her aggressive libido and that she could now experience a greater degree of mental respite, aided by the non-thinking, repetitive motions of her hand on the black crayon.

In the following session, Albertina opened a new box of crayons – albeit in a slightly less destructive manner – and she then dropped all of the contents onto the floor once again. On this occasion, she grabbed each of the remaining eleven drawing implements and then ripped off the pointed heads of each and every one in turn. I could not help but realize how much the crayons looked like penises, with their jutting tips, and as Albertina wrenched off these pointy heads, I found myself thinking about how she might well be perpetrating a symbolic attack on some dangerous phallic objects. At this juncture, I began to reflect more seriously about whether Albertina had hoped to communicate something to me about an actual experience of childhood sexual molestation. I refrained, however, from verbalizing such a direct hypothesis at this point, particularly in the absence of any further confirmatory evidence. I did, however, remark on Albertina's physical actions, and I noted, 'It looks as though you regard the heads of these crayons as very dangerous, and you seem to find it important to get rid of them.' This remark exerted a calming effect upon Albertina, who continued to produce lines on a crumpled piece of paper with this decapitated object.

Throughout the first three years of psychotherapeutic treatment, the patient drew absolutely nothing apart from a single line, either with a crayon or with a pen, and she continued to enact the same repetitive gestures, moving her hand up and down, up and down, across the page, in a soporific manner (see Figure 1.1). She would do so with such persistence that she wore out many, many boxes of crayons in the process. Indeed, every three or four weeks, I would have to replace the supply of crayons and, on each occasion, Albertina would perform the same ritual of tearing open the box and of ripping off the tips of the crayons with a tormented look in her eyes. I would invariably comment on the repetitiveness of her movements, suggesting that perhaps she derived some comfort from controlling the shape of the crayon and the movement of her arm, thus preventing anything unexpected or scary from unfolding. At times, I felt that my interpretations had become as predictable and as repetitive as Albertina's arm and hand movements.

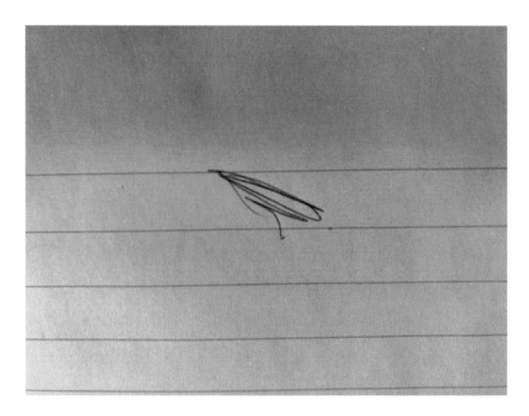

Figure 1.1 Albertina's single line drawing

Amid the third year of treatment, Albertina's drawing remained so very codified that I began to abandon any sense of hope that this woman would ever alter or enhance her obsessionally repetitive motions in any way. Fortunately, during one of our sessions, she surprised me hugely by choosing to draw not with *one* crayon of a particular colour, as she had done previously for many months but, rather, with *two* crayons of different colours, each in succession, for the very first time. She began to deploy a blue crayon and, after approximately ten minutes of doing so, she then tentatively clutched the red crayon, and produced a further, interlinking line with this new colour (see Figure 1.2). Albertina actually seemed quite pleased with what she had done, and I commented that she appeared happy to have explored something new, and to have discovered that the crayons had not harmed her in any way.

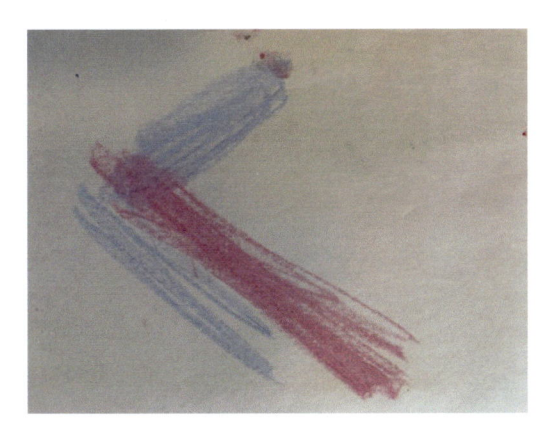

Figure 1.2 During the third year of treatment, Albertina began to draw using two colours

As the weeks unfolded, Albertina became increasingly experimental in her use of colours; and though she never digressed from her very well-entrenched habit of manufacturing a single line, she now did so in a veritable rainbow of shades. By the end of the third year of psychotherapy, the patient began to utilize not one, not two but, rather, four or five crayons of different colours for each of her pictures, all of which began to look increasingly less deadly and infinitely less barren (see Figure 1.3).

As the fourth year of treatment approached, Albertina drew a cluster of tiny little circles for the first time (see Figure 1.4). Previously, she had produced only repetitive straight lines, although in an increasingly resplendent array of colours. But the unexpected appearance of circle-shaped objects certainly marked the beginning of a potentially more vibrant chapter, which may have represented the development of new shapes and styles in her own mind and in her own life. Indeed, the creation of tiny circles, drawn in crayon, actually began to coincide with a significant diminution in her rate of spitting within the session.

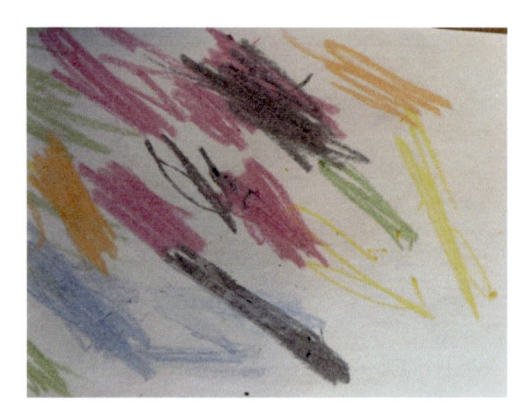

Figure 1.3 Albertina's drawing progressed to using multiple colours

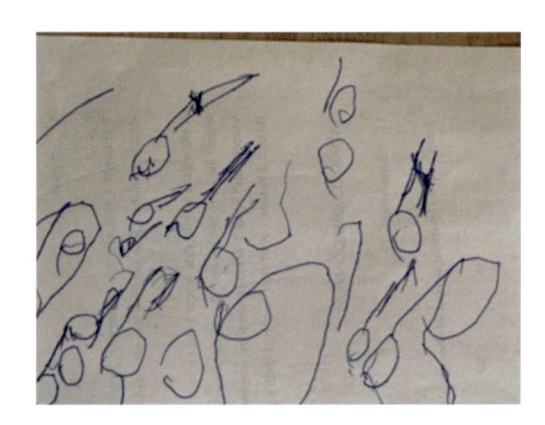

Figure 1.4 Towards the fourth year of psychotherapy, Albertina introduced circles in her drawings

In the fourth, fifth, and sixth years of psychotherapy, Albertina continued to draw both circles and lines in multiple colours, but she had not yet progressed to other pictorial configurations. She did, however, eventually conquer her anxiety about the crayons. At the outset of the sixth year of treatment, I presented Albertina with a new box, one of the many dozens that I had purchased over the long years. On this occasion, Albertina, for the very first time, actually took the crayons out of the box without ripping open the top. And though she stared intently at the drawing implements, she did not tear off the heads. Instead, she seized a blue crayon, examined it carefully in her fingertips, and then, like an ordinary, healthy child, she simply drew in a seemingly uncomplicated manner, and then grabbed several other colours as well, eventually producing a very vibrant picture (see Figure 1.5).

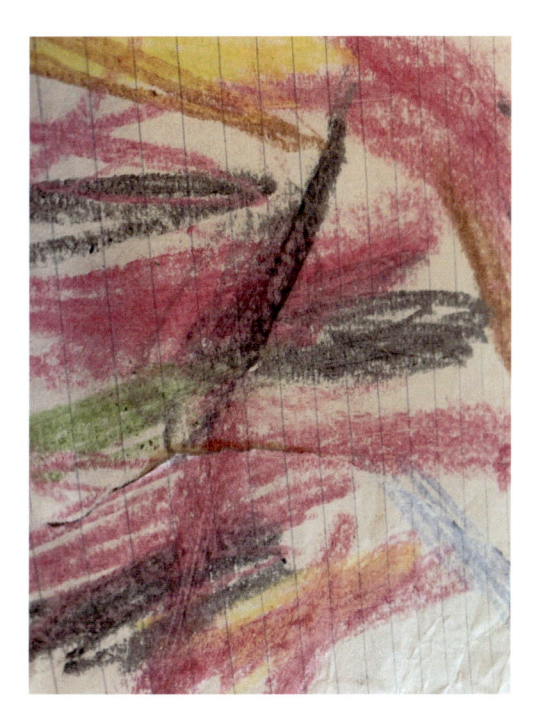

Figure 1.5 Albertina began to draw in a more relaxed way after conquering her anxiety over the crayons

Although Albertina's newfound ability to enjoy a crayon without having to destroy it may not impress any artist as a great achievement, especially after six years of work, I certainly experienced a tremendous sense of pride and accomplishment, very much akin to the feeling of observing an infant who has come to lift himself or herself up from the floor at the age of thirteen months, and who can, at long last, finally reach an object on a table. More and more, Albertina began to show evidence of making very small bite-sized strides in her ability to become better contained.

To my great delight, during the seventh and eighth years of our psychotherapeutic journey, Albertina progressed from drawing merely lines, to circles, and, finally, to creating pictures of very tiny little girls (see

Figure 1.6). I came to regard this advance as an indication that Albertina could at long last begin to develop a true sense of self with an awareness of a body.

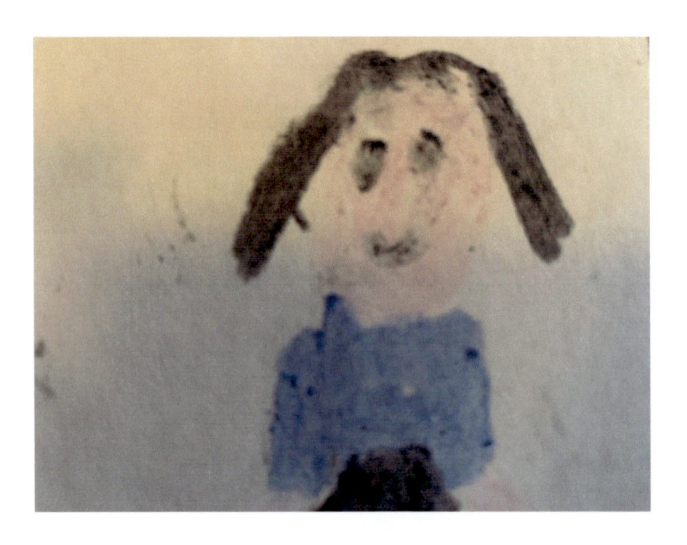

Figure 1.6 During the seventh and eighth years of psychotherapy, Albertina's drawing became figurative

3. Toileting Behaviour

Over the course of our working relationship, Albertina displayed a wide range of behaviours in relation to her use of the lavatory. In the first months of treatment, Albertina engaged in nothing untoward or inappropriate in the course of the sessions in terms of excreta. Although she spat regularly, as I have already indicated, she would never urinate or defaecate at all in the consulting room as some severely or profoundly disabled patients might do from time to time; furthermore, she never expressed a need to use the toilet at all, located down the corridor. Instead, she would arrive under escort, enter the consulting room, spit extensively, and then, after 50 minutes, would depart.

But as the treatment began to unfold, particularly in the fourth and fifth months of the first year, Albertina started to reveal other signs of being uncontained. I suspect that throughout the initial period of our weekly encounters, the patient needed to establish what sort of object I might be, and whether I would be able to tolerate her spitting behaviours

(Winnicott, 1969). But once she came to appreciate that I would, in fact, permit her to expectorate without retaliating in any way, she became much freer to demonstrate her penchant for incontinence, not only of spittle, but of urine as well.

On one particularly memorable occasion, shortly after the Easter break, Albertina entered the room as always. Within moments, she spat a stream of spittle everywhere, and then, with tremendous rapidity, she ripped off her loose-flowing caftan, and, within a matter of seconds, stood naked in the consulting room. I felt deeply concerned and, after reflecting, I responded, 'You are really trying very hard to show me that your body has never been your own, and that there have been times when anyone could have had access to your body.' Albertina did not reply to me in any obvious manner; thus, I then underscored, 'It is very important that we should try to understand this, but, first, it would be very helpful if you could put your clothes back on.' Albertina responded with surprising acquiescence and, perhaps, relief that I would not wish for her to remain so very exposed and potentially humiliated.

After Albertina put her caftan back on, she then perched on the ground and, to my amazement, she started to evacuate a stream of urine on the carpet. I explained that she might wish to use the toilet at the end of the corridor and that her escort could readily accompany her should that be of help; but Albertina simply looked at me, with an almost blank expression upon her face, and she continued to urinate, soaking a corner of the carpet. I experienced a strong sense of both nausea and irritation at that point. Calmly, I endeavoured to call upon my interpretative capacities and establish a link between these dramatic pieces of material in the session thus far, but Albertina's behaviour had attacked any capacity to think or to make links and, in consequence, I became quite resigned.

The following week, Albertina returned to my office, draped in an Indian sari, which I later learned she had inherited from an Indian patient in her residential care facility who had died two years previously. Albertina had never worn such an item of clothing previously. After entering the consulting room, Albertina lifted the hem of her sari, and then she began to stroke that part of the garment; and, to my great astonishment, she uttered her very first words. Although she struggled to speak, she did stare at me and exclaimed, 'Pretty sari, pretty sari.' I paused in my tracks and then I composed myself, commenting, 'You are showing me that you have the ability to talk to me in words, and you are excited to show me your pretty sari. This is really important. But I think you may know that the words "pretty sari" might have another meaning. Perhaps you are also telling me that you feel "pretty *sorry*" about what had happened last week, when you removed your clothing and had to urinate on the floor. You really wanted me to see how angry you can be at times and how scared you are, and how much you missed coming here for your sessions over the Easter break.' My comment seemed to evoke some small tears in Albertina's eyes. I felt cheered and hopeful that Albertina actually possessed both the capacity for speech and, also, the ability to understand homonyms and puns (namely, the difference between 'sari' and 'sorry').

As the months unfolded, Albertina would occasionally pull down her leggings in the course of our psychotherapy sessions, although she never again stripped off as she had done during the aforementioned consultation. Whenever she began to remove her leg coverings, I would ask her whether she wished to use the nearby toilet. Albertina began to nod; and, in consequence, I would open the door to the office and signal to the loyal and devoted escort who would then walk with the patient to the nearby bathroom.

Needless to say, I never accompanied Albertina to the toilet; instead, the escort did so, quite rightly. But one of my female colleagues, who worked in the office next to mine, told me that whenever my patient entered the lavatory, she always kept the door wide open, in spite of the escort's attempts to close it, thus allowing all and sundry to view her body in this more private, more vulnerable state. Perhaps Albertina wished to communicate, in yet another manner, her ongoing sense of invasion.

As the years progressed, Albertina's penchant to use the bathroom during her 50-minute sessions decreased, especially after I had begun to analyse the specific moment when she chose to indicate her wish and her need for the toilet. She would often want to urinate just before the end of the session, partly as a means of evacuating some aggressive feelings, and partly as a means of extending the length of our appointment. But, as time passed, she slowly learned to control her bladder functions and thus to use more and more of the session time productively. In the fifth year of treatment, Albertina surprised me once again. In spite of five years of refusing to allow the escort to close the door to the toilet on her behalf, Albertina eventually managed to do so on her own.

The final year of psychotherapy

After six years of regular weekly psychotherapy appointments, Albertina had undoubtedly made considerable strides. This became apparent to me on the basis of meeting with her consistently. Her sister and, also, the members of her staff team could now readily appreciate that Albertina had become much more civil and much less destructive to fellow patients and to members of the staff within her residential psychiatric facility. Prior to the onset of treatment, Albertina spat continuously, banged her head, poked her eyes, screamed, shouted, hit, and abused her fellow residents, and she masturbated, urinated, defaecated, and, in younger years, smeared menstrual blood in public. But, after more than six years of sessions, all of these symptoms had finally disappeared entirely.

The patient and I persevered with our work during the seventh and eighth years. By this point, Albertina had ceased spitting completely – a huge achievement in view of the fact that she had often spat more than 1000 times per day in her psychiatric residence and had managed as many as 200 spittles during my very first 50-minute consultation with her several years previously.

During the eighth year of our work, Albertina did spit one more time, *but only once*, in the final moments of our last session before a long Christmas break. After I interpreted that Albertina might be quite angry with me for 'abandoning' her for several weeks, she then looked regretful and turned to a box of tissues – never having done so before – and, for the very first time, she blew her nose into an ordinary Kleenex in a truly matter-of-fact fashion, just as any of our more normal-neurotic patients would have done.

At long last, Albertina had succeeded in containing her bodily fluids, especially her spittle, for perhaps the first time in her life. And those who had to interact with her could now manage to enjoy her company in a fuller way and did not need to be quite so concerned about her or, indeed, frightened that she would cover them with saliva. To my surprise and delight, the nursing staff began to invest more time and better care into Albertina, and I soon came to learn that the team would even treat her to special visits to a local hairdresser, which Albertina enjoyed immensely. The nurses would also escort her on numerous shopping trips and would, from time to time, purchase new, attractive clothing for this nearly-seventy-year-old woman; furthermore, they enrolled her in special music and art classes at a nearby charity for the handicapped. Previously, Albertina had created too much trouble for the staff, and in view of her compulsive spitting, she could not be taken into shops, or any other public places, let alone to a rehabilitation centre.

As we completed the eighth year of our work, Albertina had finally conquered her compulsive spitting entirely. She remained fully clothed, calm, and quiet, and she even stopped ripping the tips off of the crayons. She would now close the door to the lavatory and she had even begun to walk in a less chaotic manner, in spite of her advancing age and her lack of exercise. In our very final sessions, Albertina would often curl up on the psychoanalytical couch and would sometimes cover herself with the folded blanket which I kept at the foot of the divan to protect the fabric against the occasionally muddy shoes of my analysands. Although still mostly verbally silent, Albertina would, from time to time, speak in strained tones, uttering rudimentary phrases such as, 'Tuesday ... next session', or 'I want a baby ... baby, baby ...' In a sense, she had most assuredly progressed from a more paranoid-schizoid mode of functioning, wherein she feared attacks from external and internal objects, to a more depressive mode of functioning, characterized by her growing ability to mourn the loss of the idealized, fantasized life that she would probably never lead.

As our work progressed across its final stages, Albertina's spittles turned more and more into tears – a much healthier and a far more hygienic and far less aggressive style of bodily communication. Happily, as the psychotherapy unfolded, I experienced Albertina as less and less frightening and as more and more warm-hearted and loveable. Her propensity for primitive bodily communication had become transformed into a rather more psychologically mature style of relatedness. My attachment and affection towards her grew in steady stages. And I came to recognize that we both soldiered on through a very complex and unusual process together and eventually developed a greater regard and admiration for one another, having each survived a challenging set of interactions.

After eight years of regular weekly consultations, our psychotherapeutic voyage ended. I feel very proud of Albertina and her escort and her staff team for having supported this extraordinary process for so long; and I harbour much respect and gratitude to Albertina for having remained committed to this process. I believe that, in spite of her profound lifetime of handicaps, she did become more bearable and more engaging and, even, more delightful as a person.

Conclusions

Every moment of every day, all living human beings will experience an intimate relationship with saliva, as each of us retains salivary fluids in our mouth much of the time. And yet, for most individuals, this does not prove in the least bit problematic. Indeed, whenever we clean our teeth in the morning or in the evening, every one of us actually engages in a codified spitting ritual. Even Sigmund Freud would expectorate; in fact, his biographer, Dr Ernest Jones (1955, p. 410, fn. b) remarked on Freud's 'habit of hawking and spitting induced by his chronic catarrh and over-smoking.'

Babies will, of course, spit or dribble on a regular basis; but we tend to understand this as a necessary maturational phase which we endure as parents until such time as our babies learn motoric control over their salivary functions. But when a grown-up person continues to salivate as an infant does, he or she will often experience revulsion or disgust in response. We expect adult human beings to keep their fluids inside their bodies; and when they fail to do so, many of us will develop a noxious reaction.

However, in the case of severely traumatized and regressed individuals such as Albertina, the seemingly 'normal' process of spitting can actually become transformed into a type of serious psychopathology and may reach extreme and perverse dimensions wherein it becomes used not only as a means of communication, and as a method of self-protection, but, also, as a weapon against oneself and others.

Many years ago, Professor E. James Anthony, the well-known child psychoanalyst, noted that very few papers had appeared in the psychoanalytical literature about such messy topics as encopresis, for instance, owing to the sense of loathing evoked by such primitive bodily communications. As Anthony (1957, p. 157) noted, 'Clinicians on the whole, perhaps out of disgust, prefer neither to treat them nor to write about them.' Indeed, one will find many more references among the publications of psychoanalytical workers about cases involving the *retention* of bodily fluids and bodily substances such as faeces (e.g. Freud, 1905; Abraham, 1919; Sterba, 1934; Rosenfeld, 1968), than about cases consisting of the *expulsion* of substances and fluids. Indeed, the disgust and revulsion induced by patients who expectorate can often be so extreme that even the late Mrs Frances Tustin (1981, 1986), one of the boldest of British child psychotherapists, renowned for her work with severely psychotic children, mentioned to me, during an interview, that she would simply terminate the treatment of any child who spat in her face (Kahr, 1994).

Dr Sigmund Freud (1900a) did, of course, write about the expulsion of urine as a manifestation of masculinity and penetrativeness in his magnum opus *Die Traumdeutung*; and his German disciple, Dr Karl Abraham, studied the sadistic aspects of excretion in his psychoanalytical essay on ejaculatio praecox (Abraham, 1917; cf. Abraham, 1920). Some more modern workers in the field have written about expulsion and soiling (e.g. Shane, 1967; Flynn, 1987; Forth, 1992), but very few have shared their thoughts about saliva per se. Dr Bertram Lewin (1930), the noted American psychoanalyst, did produce a classic paper about smearing (cf. Sinason, 1992). But, on the whole, the primitivity and infantility of spitting has remained relatively untheorized, for very understandable reasons.

Mr Paul Barrows (1996), a British child psychotherapist who had worked in the NHS, published a very helpful clinical report on youngsters who soil, which may have some relevance to the problem of spitting. Barrows explained that soiling by child patients might be understood as an attempt to control an object; more specifically, he came to regard the act of soiling as a defence against an oedipal coupling. In other words, when the child envies the exclusivity of parental intercourse (cf. Money-Kyrle, 1971), he or she will soil as a means of attacking the parental couple by intruding into the privacy of the relationship between the mother and the father. In other words, once the child has urinated or defaecated, one of the parents must then help clean the youngster's body; and, in this way, the little boy or little girl will have succeeded in engaging in a relationship with an adult caregiver, thus interrupting the potentiality of any parental sexual intercourse.

As we will recall, during the sixth year of psychotherapy, Albertina had not spat for weeks and weeks, and yet, on one particular occasion, I happened to sneeze. Immediately thereafter, Albertina produced spittle for the very first time in ages, ostensibly as a means of interrupting my private congress – my private *intercourse* – with my own sneeze.

I suspect that, more generally, whenever Albertina spat, she did so for a multiplicity of reasons:
1. As a means of communicating internal states of distress and disorientation and traumatization;
2. As a means of conveying that she had suffered from possible

sexual trauma, evidenced by her use of saliva as a fluid which she inserted into her ears and into her vagina and anus;
3. As a means of discharging sadistic libidinal strivings, and as a means of attacking a hated object in fantasy;
4. As a means of interrupting an oedipal coupling which could provoke terrific enviousness.

The psychology of spitting remains a very unexamined area in the fields of psychoanalysis and psychotherapy. I trust that these preliminary observations about the role of infantile-like spitting – a deeply powerful form of primitive bodily communication – will help to shed a certain amount of light upon this highly vexing and potentially very destructive symptom.

The analysis of a piece of psychotherapeutic work remains quite a complicated undertaking. So many psychoanalytical writers have pontificated about the effective ingredients in psychological work, ranging from the mutative role of transference interpretations (e.g. Strachey, 1934), to the provision of a secure clinical framework (e.g. Langs, 1973). Although the creation of a setting in which reliable treatment can unfold, accompanied by the proffering of intelligent and thoughtful interpretations, will always remain foundational to the practice of psychoanalytical work, one must not underestimate the importance of simply *surviving* the experience, a feature highlighted by Dr Donald Winnicott (1962, 1969), and of *containing* the distress of the patient, a crucial undercurrent emphasised by Dr Wilfred Bion (1962a, 1962b). I remain grateful to Dr Susanna Isaacs Elmhirst, who had worked with both Winnicott and Bion, and who had served as the clinical supervisor to this case over several years, for recalling that each of these iconic men had deployed the phrase 'white heat' (quoted in Elmhirst, 1996), quite independently, to describe the experience of treating patients who had the capacity to create a very intense, even frightening, clinical encounter (cf. Elmhirst, 1981). This 'white heat' must be survived, and it must be contained; and, in many respects, I regard the containment of the potent affects which emerged in the treatment of Albertina as one of the most crucial elements of the psychotherapeutic adventure.

Based upon his extensive clinical experiences with individual psychotic patients and, also, upon his wartime work with groups of soldiers, Bion developed a theory about the role of containment of psychic material by the parent (and, also, by the psychoanalyst) as a means of detoxifying and defusing the dangerousness of the powerful affects at hand. Bion (1970, p. 95) noted that, 'an object is placed into a container in such a way that either the container or the contained object is destroyed.' But if the container proves sufficiently robust, then both participants will survive in a more fruitful way (cf. Hinshelwood, 1989).

Although continuously tempted to terminate the treatment of Albertina because of the oftentimes unbearable psychical burden of sitting with this highly pained woman for so many alternately crazed and silent sessions, I nonetheless refrained from doing so, supported by good internal and external objects in my own professional sphere (e.g. personal psychoanalysis, clinical supervision, training, coursework, collegial support, and so forth). Having survived the 'white heat' of Albertina's attacks and projections, she and I managed to progress through to a more bearable state, in which this troubled woman could experience greater inner peace, increasingly secure in the knowledge that both she and I would live to witness the end of the session.

In this report, I have attempted to demonstrate the ways in which a knowledge of psychoanalytical ideas, influenced by exposure to the skills of infant observation (e.g. Winnicott, 1941; Bick, 1964) and to disability psychotherapy (e.g. Sinason, 1992), can enhance our capacity to study non-verbal patients in great detail, and thus develop a richer toleration of non-verbal behaviour and, moreover, a fuller ability to understand its meaning. Although many had once questioned the utility of psychoanalytical approaches to the treatment of the handicapped (e.g. Scharff and Scharff, 1992), more recent writings have suggested that ongoing dynamic insights may prove quite useful in the rehabilitation of those who suffer from extraordinary liabilities and disadvantages (e.g. Sinason, 1992, 1999, 2012; Corbett, Cottis, and Morris, 1996; Hollins, 1997, 2002; Hollins and Sinason, 2000; Blackman, 2003; Wilson, 2003; Cottis, 2009, 2017; Curen, 2009, 2018; Corbett, 2014, 2018; Frankish, 2016; Kahr, 2017, 2021a, 2021b).

Classical psychoanalysis and classical psychotherapy can, in fact, provide patients with an opportunity to transform their projectile spitting and other forms of violent attacks into a much more contained posture. Likewise, one may even facilitate the development of rudimentary language among our more verbally impaired patients (cf. Tirelli, 1989).

It will be my hope that, in time, Albertina and other patients who have struggled with similar disabilities and with comparable traumata will become better able to hurl words of abuse in their psychotherapy sessions, as a means of communicating and working-through earlier painful experiences and cruel injustices, so that both they, and their families and carers, will ultimately derive greater satisfaction from their lives. By transforming primitive bodily communications into more sophisticated verbal communications (whether conveyed through words or through crayons), we continue to have the privilege of facilitating the growth of the healthy human mind.

ACKNOWLEDGEMENTS

I wish to express my deepest thanks and appreciation to Ms Raffaella Hilty, the most gracious of editors, for her warm invitation to contribute a more extensive version of this case history and for her boldness in tackling the difficult topic of 'primitive bodily communication'. Ms Hilty offered many helpful comments about this essay. Likewise, I owe immense thanks to Dr Valerie Sinason for having kindly read this chapter in great detail.

I could not have undertaken such lengthy psychotherapeutic work without the tremendous support and wisdom which I received from so many truly wise teachers, including the late Dr Abrahão Brafman, Dr Bernard Barnett, the late Dr Murray Cox, the late Dr Susanna Isaacs Elmhirst, Profesora Estela Welldon and Dr Gianna Williams. Dr Valerie Sinason offered regular, immense and unparalleled supervisory enlightenment over many decades and served as my teacher, my boss, and my inspiration. I had the privilege to work with Dr Sinason in both the Tavistock Clinic Mental Handicap Team and the Tavistock Clinic Mental Handicap Workshop and certainly could not have facilitated this treatment without her pioneering insights. I thank many of my former disability colleagues from the early 1990s including Dr Sheila Bichard, the late Mrs Sandra Linford, Mrs Judy Townley, Mrs Judith Usiskin, and Dr Sarah Wynick.

I had the privilege of discussing this case with colleagues at the Tavistock Clinic in London on many occasions, and at numerous other institutions as well, over the years, and I convey my warm gratitude to the many audience members who helped me to process this difficult material. Earlier incarnations of this case history appeared in the journals *American Imago: Psychoanalysis and the Human Sciences* (Kahr, 2005,

2008), published by the Johns Hopkins University Press of Baltimore, Maryland; the *British Journal of Psychotherapy* (Kahr, 2017, 2019), published by John Wiley and Sons of Hoboken, New Jersey; and *Body, Movement and Dance in Psychotherapy: An International Journal for Theory, Research and Practice* (Kahr, 2021b), published by Routledge/ Taylor & Francis Group of London and Abingdon, Oxfordshire; and *The International Journal of Forensic Psychotherapy* (Kahr, 2021c), published by Phoenix Publishing House of Bicester, Oxfordshire. I crafted other shortened versions as well in two of my solo-authored books, *Bombs in the Consulting Room: Surviving Psychological Shrapnel* (Kahr, 2020a) and *On Practising Therapy at 1.45 A.M.: Adventures of a Clinician* (Kahr, 2020b), both published by Routledge/Taylor & Francis Group of London and Abingdon, Oxfordshire, and in one edited book on *Shattered States: Disorganised Attachment and its Repair. The John Bowlby Memorial Conference Monograph 2007*, originally released by Karnac Books of London (Kahr, 2012). I extend my appreciation to the editors of those essays and to the publishers of those full-length texts. I offer my very deepest thanks to Ms Susannah Frearson, Senior Editor at Routledge – part of the Taylor & Francis Group – and to her colleagues, for their tremendous helpfulness in so many regards.

The current version represents not only an amalgamation and rewriting of my previous essays and chapters but, moreover, a fuller expansion, crafted with the benefit of much hindsight and further time for reflection. I extend my warm gratitude to our inspiring and visionary Publisher at Karnac Books, Dr Stephen Setterberg, and to the hugely accomplished Publishing Team, for facilitating the production of this important edited book, including Mr Richard Atienza-Hawkes, Ms Vicky Capstick, Mr Patrick Dawson, Ms Christina Wipf Perry, Dr Kathy Rooney, Ms Jane Ryan, Ms Alice Waterfall, Ms Liz Wilson, and Ms Emily Wootton.

Notes

1. The original German phrase reads: 'Schwerer Fall' (Jung, 1906a, p. 7).
2. The original German sentence reads: 'Es ist nichts Seltenes, daß kleine Kinder die Hand dessen, der sie trägt, beschmutzen' (Freud, 1906a, p. 8).
3. The original German sentence reads: 'Sein Spucken ist Sperma-Ejakulation' (Freud, 1908a, p. 75).
4. The original German phrase reads: 'Aus dem Buben wird nichts werden' (quoted in Freud, 1900a, p. 149).
5. I have elected to refer to the young boy by his birth name, Sigismund Freud, rather than as Sigmund Freud, as he had not changed his identity until later in life.
6. The original German sentence reads: 'Anna speit Feuer, wenn der Name Rank genannt wird' (Freud, 1924, p. 362). As the correspondence between Professor Sigmund Freud and Dr Max Eitingon has not appeared in the English language, I have provided my own translation.

CHAPTER 2

Working with primitive bodily communications in the context of unbearable trauma in non-verbal patients

Smell, silence, and Winnie the Pooh

Valerie Sinason

'Thou hast no hands to wipe away thy tears, nor tongue to
tell me who hath martyr'd thee'
Shakespeare *Titus Andronicus*, 3,1 106–7

This chapter will provide an overview of work with intellectual disability and extreme trauma when working with non-verbal patients. Talking treatment works even when it is the body and mind in the body that communicate. Child psychotherapy training, with its focus on baby and toddler observations, privileges the body countertransference and understanding of preverbal states. It is not surprising that a significant number of child psychotherapists have also completed an adult training in order to work with those of all ages with profound multiple intellectual disabilities. This chapter will focus on patients with no verbal speech, whose only communication could come through bodily behaviours such as head banging, defecating and bleeding.

This subject is rarely spoken about. We have bodies with orifices – us human animals – and we need to empty out urine and faeces. Sometimes mucous comes from our noses, blood from menstruation or wounds, semen, vaginal fluid, breast milk, vomit and dribble from our mouths. We know this and we disavow it. We find it hard in the West to have a body. And all over the world all religions and cultures find different aspects of bodies unbearable. When substances leave the body and decay they frighten us by telling us about mortality and in some cultures become fetish items – nail clippings, pubic hair, menstrual blood. To face these unpopular, rarely spoken of subjects, means going back in our memories to earliest childhood, or to our preverbal memories that can lie hidden in our bodies. These memories are also socially and culturally embedded. Let me take you there first.

A loving mother prepared the bath for her tiny baby. She checked the water with her elbow. She had a fluffy towel with hood already on her lap. The room temperature was optimum as she lovingly washed and cradled the tiny baby. There was a sudden moment where she roughly wiped his mouth with the flannel. The baby gave a newborn falling reflex movement and cried and she quickly comforted him. He was soothed and for a moment I thought I had imagined that moment. The same thing happened the following week. When the baby was three months old, the moment the flannel touched his mouth he laughed. 'Oh you like it do you,' said the mother jovially, as if recognizing the aggression in that micro-moment. From then on it became a moment of play. Later work was able to show the mother's fear of greediness and dirt in which she could not bear the thought of any extra residue on the baby's mouth having contact with her nipple. She realized this was likely to have been what she experienced at the breast. This was a micro-moment amongst hours of loving care and the baby boy turned into a healthy loving boy and young man. What happens when the balance alters?

In preparing this chapter I had a sudden memory from over 50 years ago when I was a trainee infant school teacher. Little Marie (not her real name), anxiously approached me before morning register in the infant school top class. 'Miss, Miss,' she whispered urgently. 'There's a rude book in the library and I picked it up but I don't know if my mum will be cross with me.' With tears building up in her eyes she passed me a worn-down copy of that perennial favourite, Winnie the Pooh. Pooh. Poo. The dirty word, the powerful word, the Voldemort word, too delicious and terrifying to contemplate. It was a word that could provoke explosive guffaws of laughter, or whispered giggles and secret smiles, like 'farts' or 'knickers' or evoke terror and shame. It was resonant of the particular horror in the reception class at the thought of not managing to last out a day in big school without 'an accident'. Every good infant school I knew had a cupboard generously filled with spare knickers, pants, trousers and skirts in case of such accidents. What genius of A. A. Milne to create such a name and spelling! But poor Marie came from a particular cultural and religious background that was strong on badness and reading a book with a title like that might be seen as immoral. How I broached this for Marie and her mother is at the end of this chapter. However, what I wanted to follow through here was how our early attitudes to and experiences of feeding and defecating impact on us throughout the life cycle. From the same period, another memory was unlocked. When I took a group of infant school children to the zoo for their special summer outing there was something that made all the adults sick and disgusted. You could see the horror on their faces and the downward curves of disgust on their lips. At the same time, this was something which delighted all the children. In fact it was the highlight of their visit. The chimpanzees were defecating, catching a stool with their hands and picking it up to eat. What price does toilet training come with or evolutionary warnings about disease to turn this narcissistic delight into hate, shame and disgust?

Two-year-old Dennis was sitting on a potty. He produced a stool. 'Well done, what a big clever boy,' said his mother proudly. Dennis toddled up to examine it. 'Looks like big brown chocolate sausage,' he chortled with glee. Little Susan sniffed her potty with appreciation. 'Look what I made, lovely smell,' she boasted. These are the moments of normal pleasure at creativity and mastery. Before the fall ... which seems to last a lifetime for many.

When working with mothers of babies I found that whilst most could get used to the smell of their own baby's faeces, the smell of other babies' faeces filled them with disgust. When providing occasional babysitting for each other, the thought of changing nappies of another baby felt difficult. And even the mothers who usually had no problem changing their own baby's nappies felt more negatively if the Babygro was suddenly soaked with explosive diarrhoea with the contents covering their hands. Could this be an evolutionary fear of infection added to shame? Or a re-awareness of the smells that distinguish me from not-me? Babies of just a few weeks old can turn their head to the side of a pillow where their mother's breast milk has been placed. The role of smell in defining me and not-me can be found in some of the origins of racism, a discrimination that is potentially useful that has somehow become twisted in some homes and cultures. We need to consider our thoughts and feelings openly here as it is intrinsic to our clinical work. The toddler and small child's omnipotent delight in producing a faecal baby coming from their bottom, surpassing the acts of creation provided by mother, somehow transforms through toilet training. The omnipotence needs to be worked through for future healthy development but the casualties can be high. There are myriad daily tragedies in which otherwise loving parents who praise their child's development of self-agency in toileting revert to acting out their own preverbal traumas by becoming punitive and shaming when accidents happen. In homes with love and a good-enough attachment there can still be internalized shame at the fear of an accident – going right through into adult life.

Tragically, institutions can re-enact group traumas by restricting the right of children to go to the toilet when they need to, or by limiting the amount of toilet paper they can have. It is worth noting that soft toilet paper, which we take for granted in most of the UK, was only introduced into the workplace during the Second World War as women in the workplace complained about the thin hard paper! It is interesting to note that the panic buying at the start of Covid throughout the West was predominantly for toilet paper. Whilst anal hygiene is essential both for the individual body and the danger of pathogens for others, it seemed to many of us that the panic came from more shame and fear-based origins. Cleaning the anus after defecation is accomplished by toilet paper in most Western countries and with that comes not only a higher standard of living but also a fear of gaining closer contact with a 'dirty' area. Although China used toilet paper in the second century BC and Rabelais spoke of its ineffectiveness in the sixteenth century, in terms of Western culture, Joseph Gayetty invented modern toilet paper in New York in 1857 and most Western countries followed.

The majority of countries in the world do not have toilet paper either for standard of living reasons or for culture, which has had to incorporate what is possible. Without money for toilet paper, attempts to install modern flush toilets can be rendered useless as pages from newspapers or other materials found will not flush. Cleaning the anus with water and with the left hand in some cultures has also added to the stigma about left-handedness which still remains. Whether there is probably and possibly an evolutionary need for shame to be instilled in order to prevent infection, which exacerbates the impact of internalized shame and punishment, we can see the tragic fact that cross-culturally concentration camps all over the world deprive their victims of faecal autonomy as a first and major step in humiliating and objectifying them.

I am initially focusing on shared human biological imperatives as to work with those with severe physical or intellectual disabilities, the very young or the very old, means facing these memories and thoughts in ourselves. This vulnerability over our animal waste links the very young and the very old. In a poem written about visiting an old peoples' home in 'Over and Out' (*Nightshift*, 1995) I wrote:

Filipino assistants are disinfecting the floors
Scrubbing at shadows of loss and incontinence
While the owners of the shadows
Are wheeled into the garden
To dry

The Island of Leros in Greece became notorious in the 1980s and 1990s. Before the world learned of the terrible conditions Romanian orphans lived in, Leros showed us how we treat 'disposable' people. The island had a tragic history. It had been a leper colony, then the Greek colonels sent their communist prisoners there and then the mentally ill and intellectually disabled, who had not been visited for over six months, were sent there. It was an island, symbolically and literally. Patients died from being fed pureed food lying down. Men and women lost the use of their limbs through being tied to beds. There were few words. A courageous Greek psychiatrist, Dr Jon Tsiantis, who was also a psychotherapist, went to the European Commission to gain help to improve the lot of the islanders. When I was invited to go to the island, as part of a European Commission attempt to provide therapeutic help, I went to Professor Israel Kolvin to ask for advice. He was a professor of psychiatry who came to work at the Tavistock Clinic in London. He went on the first official visit to Leros. When I asked how I should prepare for my visit he had succinct two-word advice, 'Think shit!' And that was what I did. When I arrived at the island sparkling by the sea I was asked by the psychologists meeting me if I would like a tour to see how beautiful it was. But I couldn't. I needed to follow my advice and go straight to the wards in the stark hospital buildings.

Through the poems I wrote on Leros (Sinason, 1995, p. 68) we find how the advice had been internalized.

(b)
A patient carries the dirty washing
Each morning he walks up the cold steps
With a sack of shit
Like Sisyphus

(c)

Patients lie in their bed-silences
Fed lying down with pureed food
No drinks, no cups, no cutlery
No sanitary towels no toilets
No books, no visits, no outings
Everything leaks

(d)
'You can do anything on an island,' said Circe
Turning men to pigs

(e)
In the morning the smell is of urine
In the evening the shit smell spreads
One untrained woman is on duty
Ward after ward after ward with dim lights
And nothing

5 b) Rehabilitation
The children come in one by one
They bring the ward smell with them
The new world is linked to the old
By urine
The patients mark the territory like dogs
They return as children

When I entered the first ward I had prepared a greeting in Greek, 'Hello, my name is Valerie and I come from London.' I stood facing the appalling sight of people treated as disposable, several on iron beds tied together. No separate lockers, no private property, no adequate clothes. I wanted to run away. In my head I silently said to myself, 'If you do not go and talk to someone here I will never speak to you again,' – a rare kind of splitting! I walked to an entangled group to say my sentence and a young man with Down's syndrome somehow extricated his body from what felt like a living communal grave. I held my hand out and he shook it. Then I slowly said goodbye and walked out, the eyes following me from all the cold iron beds with their huddled occupants. I walked out and into the bathroom and scrubbed and scrubbed and scrubbed at my hands. I felt sick and tearful … The societally unwanted, those with severe intellectual disability are treated like waste that needs to be flushed away, disposed of. They were the first victims of Nazism and in almost all cultures they are the put away, secreted, disposed of so that polite society can continue not thinking nature produces diversity. To deprive people of faecal agency and to leave them malnourished physically and emotionally turns them into an unbearable shadow image we do not want to get close to. With Leros, I was seeing humans hibernating from their richness and knowledge because it was not safe to think or know anything.

One year later I visited again and the first group of patients had been moved to a hostel in Athens, the first hostel for disabled people in Greece. When I rang the doorbell the man with Down's syndrome greeted me warmly. He wore a shirt and trousers and looked so proud and sentient. It was heart warming to see the human resilience. Followed by an interpreter he showed me his small private clean room. There was a wardrobe, chair, bed and desk. He opened the wardrobe. He had two pairs of trousers and two shirts in it. He was so proud. His actions spoke volumes. There was no need for words. He pointed to the room with wonderment. We both remembered him tied into a shared stark bed. Then in the group for all those survivors of Leros he said to me, through the translator, with warmth and intelligence shining on his face, 'I remember you. You held my hand. In Leros.'

In this time of Covid we know the wariness of touch. But this was a different wariness. It was the fear of touching the unclean other, the objectified other, the projected-into destroyed other. In this context I was part of the dissembling world, the part of the world free to travel and speak and be heard, a world built on as well as adjacent to the silence of sufferers. This extreme example, where I had to face my fear of the othered, helped me later in differentiating countertransference that came from the other's projection into me, activating feelings in me and what was my problem alone. Countertransference helps us understand the meaning behind the communication. Skip the paragraphs about Maureen and Ali if you cannot bear more faecal examples. This is painful material.

Here is Maureen. She had no verbal speech. She was 19 with multiple abandonments. She had blinded herself in one eye with her eye poking, had caused a collapsed rectum with her anal poking and smeared faeces and menstrual blood on the walls of her room. I have written extensively about her elsewhere (Sinason, 2010) but not this episode. Maureen came into the room early in treatment looking furious. Her worker had told me how exhausted staff were, putting her to bed in a clean room and seeing shit smeared on the walls in the morning. They had no night waking staff. It took time to clean. Maureen clearly felt shamed by this. Inside the room I commented on how hard it must be for her hearing people talk about her without the power to tell them to stop. I wondered if she felt her privacy had been invaded as she had not told me herself but her worker had. She nodded. She looked at me angrily and then a sadistic smile spread across her face and lifting her tunic top she pulled off her wet incontinence pad and moved her wheelchair nearer to me. In my mind I could guess she was going to defecate in the room and felt horrified. Feeling invaded as she must so often, in slow motion I watched as a large turd was carefully aimed onto the clinic's new carpet with her raising herself in her chair so that she was not affected by it at all. I found it hard to speak. In my mind I was saying, 'Don't run your wheelchair over that …' I watched mute as with a great smile she wheeled her chair over and over it. The smell was awful and the new institutional hard-wearing carpet was thoroughly soiled. I had not wanted the carpet because of body fluids in such work and here was my worst fear coming true. There was a paralyzed silence. As I prepared to find my voice and speak, her smile went and she looked frightened. I said she might feel like a piece of shit and furious at having her privacy breached by her staff and furious that I had been a shit to listen to the staff member. But I could not think with this smell and mess in the room and now I needed to clean it before I could speak. I also said I needed to open the window. For almost the whole session with disinfectant and water and reams of kitchen roll I cleared the mess. She just listened with a serious face as I wondered aloud about her actions. I said many things. How hard it must be to have staff to clean her and toilet her, to not have body privacy, to be spoken about … how shitty it must feel. But now my room and me had been treated like shit.

She never did that again. She experienced a momentary secondary gain at making a lucky human feel invaded and shitty and helpless but she cared enough about attachment and linking to work that through.

Ali, aged ten, with a severe intellectual disability, had been anally gang-raped by a group of men. His sexual re-enactments with the dolls in the room was unbearable as it felt so literal. However, the rawness and savagery of the experiences he had gone through could not be expressed adequately in that semi-symbolic way. He pulled his trousers down and stuck a pen up his anus hole, making sexual noises. Taking the biro out, covered with faeces, he licked it lasciviously saying, 'Lovely lovely.' I felt sick. I could not remove the biro from him without being involved in abuse so I felt a nauseous collusive witness. I wondered aloud about the poor little boy Ali who had to witness big boys and men hurting him. He was so clever he managed to find a way of calling it exciting but it didn't work because it made him feel sick. And I felt sick watching just like little Ali might have. He went to the sink and gargled and washed his mouth.

Working with victims of cult abuse, many had been forced to eat faeces. It had been a deliberate attempt to make them feel beyond normal human etiquette and ways of being. They were terrified of touch and longing for it but felt profoundly contaminated. It was also another way of silencing them. Who would want to be with them? Just as in Leros, I found that it mattered to hold a hand (with consent of course) when an experience of eating faeces was described or mimed or drawn.

Let me move now from such particularly unbearable descriptions. Outside of abuse, what the babies, the very old and infirm and the profoundly multiply disabled share is the involuntary defaecating, urinating and dribbling. I do not consider it surprising that working with the very old and the very young carries less status. Whilst we understand the impact of attachment patterns on how we deal with extreme dependency in the young and the old, we are rarely asked to examine the impact of the non-verbal, the impact of orifices, smell, faeces, urine, saliva, sperm, menstrual blood, the unwashed on work status. I realized as a young infant school teacher that there was an implicit career hierarchy linked to the age of client you worked with. As an infant school teacher I had less status (and salary) than when later lecturing in a sixth form college or university even though the infant school work was more demanding, and, arguably, had the greatest long-term effect on the hopes, aspirations and impact on the pupil. As a child psychotherapist I had less status than when I qualified as an adult psychoanalyst. From babyhood to young adults the status markers slowly rise, only to sink again when working with the severely disabled or the elderly, the age I am now! I will not forget the senior adult psychoanalyst who, after I presented work with a patient with multiple intellectual and physical disabilities, said, critically, 'But this is only just like being a mother!', managing to insult mothers, the disabled and disability therapy in one simple sentence. We can also note the regular and insidious negatives received by the woman (particularly) or man who stays at home whilst their child/children are young and the deprecating 'just' a housewife!

As a young mother at home in the 1960s I had a poem 'Cabbage Liberation' published in the now defunct *Nova* magazine. It began

'And what do YOU do in the day'
They ask
Dragging me live and kicking
To the cabbage patch
In a shroud of Kleenex
Anointed with Dettol'.

It rather mirrors the discussions with retired elderly people that include, barely hidden under the surface, 'What did you do when you were a proper person?'

In working with children and adults with profound multiple disabilities, extreme abuse, homelessness, all smells are experienced acutely and you need to know that with all the analysis in the world there are some smells or acts that are not bearable to us. For example, as a child and adult psychotherapist I have dealt with blood, semen, urine, faeces, dribbling in the therapy room but what has disturbed me most, regardless of the intention of the other, was the other wiping snot from their nose and eating it. No analysis made any difference. I just had to accept that for whatever early reasons I could not bear it. As an infant school teacher doing exercises with the class was the worst moment, when saying, 'Breathe in, breath out' brought all the nasal sound effects and sights I could not bear! I just needed lots of boxes of tissues.

What can we hear? What can we see? What can we smell? What can we feel? Trauma can accentuate all senses. A painting, a book, a shape, a colour, something the therapist wears can feel like a missile to the traumatized patient. And we can watch the regurgitation of dribble, smell it together with the seeping of urine. This work enters us at a deep sensory level and when change happens it is dramatic and wonderful.

Marie's parents came for a special meeting as I wanted to show them Marie's pictures and how well her writing was coming on. I said I had high hopes for Marie. 'Poo to that,' said her father dismissively, but hiding a secret delighted smile. 'Language!' said Marie's mother embarrassedly. I was delighted. The key had been given to me. 'Ah,' I said, 'so that's where she gets it from.' 'What?' they both asked. I said there was a very famous book for children, they might have heard of it. Winnie the Pooh. About a bear. It was a story children loved having read to them and really helped them learn. Little Marie wanted to learn and get a book from the library but she was worried it was a bad book because it had that word in it. 'Oh, the little lamb,' said Mother softly and happily. Father just smiled. When Marie joined us her mother patted her head and said she was a good girl to check on books with her teacher and she could read any book in the library her teacher let her read.

CHAPTER 3

The sound of silence: working with people with an intellectual disability who self-harm

David O'Driscoll

All patients referred to are fictitious composites but are based on clinical material encountered during my work as a psychotherapist for the National Health Service.

When I first started working in the NHS in 1999, I had only recently qualified as a psychotherapist. Despite many years of support work in intellectual disability (ID) services (O'Driscoll, 2019), I had only the briefest experience working therapeutically with this group, during a short placement. In fact, my main psychotherapy training did not have any lectures or seminars on working with a person with an intellectual disability, a situation sadly still the case today as I write this in January 2021. So when my manager allocated a new referral to me, a 47-year-old non-verbal woman with moderate intellectual disabilities, for 'bereavement counselling for the loss of her mother', my first thought was that this would be a consultation for the staff. I would support them to support her, rather than work directly with her. There was not a great deal of personal information about Ms A, although what there was, was a rather startling statement about her, 'biting her hand, eye-poking, scratching her arms, to such an extent it was bleeding heavily', and on one occasion, while 'visiting the day centre kitchen, she had started hitting her head with a saucepan'. Ms A had also, at another time, hit a service user. The staff reported that this was very much out of character. The referral from the GP had requested 'bereavement counselling', while the social worker had suggested 'a behaviour modification program of some sort or failing that maybe some music therapy?'

This chapter will explore ways of working with people with an intellectual disability who use their body to communicate their internal distress. I will first discuss what an intellectual disability is, the accompanying vulnerability to trauma and how it can help explain why people attack their bodies. Then I will look at the therapeutic treatment of self-harm in this population and how I worked with Ms A. I will also draw on my experience of working with other service users via a couple of vignettes. The innovative work of Valerie Sinason, who is the main influence behind what today we would term as 'disability therapy' (Kahr, 2000), will be discussed.

What is intellectual disability?

People with intellectual disabilities are a heterogeneous group. The severity of intellectual disability differs widely. At one end of the spectrum, people with mild intellectual disability merge into the general population; this is the biggest group, forming around 95 per cent of those with intellectual disability. People in the other two categories – moderate and severe – are more likely to have contact with support services and are potentially more likely to be non-verbal too. Severely intellectually disabled people may function at the level of infants and be unable to feed themselves or sit unaided and be doubly incontinent. The causes of their disability also vary. Some intellectual disabilities are associated with genetic abnormalities such as Down's syndrome, others with poisoning in utero (foetal alcohol syndrome, for example), or birth trauma. For the most part, however, and particularly with less severely disabled people, the causes are unclear. Genetic factors and aspects of the childhood environment may well play a part. If there is no organic brain damage, trauma can be an actual cause of the intellectual disability – for example, due to abuse or violence, parental substance abuse, or poverty in the home. Not everybody with an intellectual disability will need a specialist support service. Those who do will come under the remit of a NHS multidisciplinary team, most often comprising health professionals such as psychiatrists, nurses and speech and occupational therapists. The psychotherapeutic options are limited – generally teams offer clinical psychologists, who focus on behavioural approaches, or creative therapists. There are very few counsellors or psychotherapists working in such teams or specializing in this field.

I work as a psychoanalytic psychotherapist four days a week, running clinics where I see around 12 clients a week. The majority are in the mid intellectual disability range, but I also see a few people who are non-verbal. Interestingly, my team tends to assume I can only work with people who are verbal and are surprised when I say I can also work with those who are non-verbal. There is a tendency to refer individuals for a creative therapy approach, such as music therapy, or introduce a behaviour modification plan for the support staff in the majority of cases.

There is a phrase we use in intellectual disabilities services, that people who are non-verbal 'do not use words to communicate'. The causes are not always understood; for various reasons they have not developed the capacity to speak. It is clearly linked to their learning disability and the majority are in the severe category. However, it is rare. It is different from mutism, which is when someone chooses not to speak for whatever reason. These clients use a wide repertoire of non-verbal behaviours to communicate their needs, wishes and emotions to carers and professionals, such as facial expression, gesticulation and non-verbal utterances. Given how much human communication relies on the spoken word, it is not surprising that they are very vulnerable to being misinterpreted and misunderstood and present considerable challenges for support workers. Phelvin (2012) highlighted their vulnerability to being misinterpreted and the challenges for support workers to develop a good relationship, or use their intuition.

Mental health, intellectual disability and trauma

The need for psychological support in this group is evident. For example, we know that people with ID are vulnerable to the effects of loss, and are four times more likely to have mental health issues than the general population (Cooper et al., 2007). They are vulnerable to abuse, trauma and bullying (i.e. Brown, Stein and Tuck, 1995; O'Driscoll, 2015). Historically, people with intellectual disabilities have been devalued and have faced significant discrimination and disadvantage, and this has not changed much, if at all, today (Jarrett, 2020).

The evidence that people with intellectual disability are particularly vulnerable to trauma has somewhat belatedly shown a developing interest in finding psychotherapeutic ways to help them. In part this is due to the pioneering work of the psychoanalyst Valerie Sinason. She argues that traumatic symptoms are significantly under-recognized in people with intellectual disability. She has also observed from her clinical work how the disability itself is experienced as a trauma: 'Opening your eyes ... to the realization that you will not be an Austen, Einstein, Madonna or Picasso can be painful enough to the ordinary adolescent. Opening your eyes to admitting you look, sound, walk, talk, move or think differently from the ordinary, average person ... takes greater reserves of courage, honesty and toleration of one's envy.' (Sinason, 1992, p. 20). One of Sinason's very important concepts is the 'handicapped smile' – the fixed grin worn by many people with intellectual disabilities. This, she argues, often hides trauma; it is used to create a fiction of a happy self to keep people around them happy with them: 'People who are close to grief and cannot bear it encourage happiness and smiling' (Sinason, 1992, p. 119). What is of particular concern is that, despite Sinason's work, many services may be superficially aware of trauma but have little understanding of the treatment options or its long-term effects. Sinason has written, 'I learned for psychotherapy to work there had to be the possibility of the actual impairment itself being able to be verbalised and thought about. I also learned how self-injury in some children and adults could represent a "secondary handicap" – a displacement activity that covers up the fear and the shame around the original difference.' (Sinason, 1992, p. 97).

Self-harm and intellectual disabilities

For many practitioners working in intellectual disability services, self-harm is a complex, disturbing and often upsetting issue. The literature on people with intellectual disability who self-harm is dominated by behavioural or biological approaches (Heslop and Lovell, 2013). The biological approach focuses on the idea that self-harm is caused by illness, injury, chemical imbalances in the brain or seizure activity, or is genetic. This clearly can be a factor. For example, the person may have an undiagnosed medical condition or may be in pain and cannot express this in words and may use self-harm to distract themselves from the symptoms. 'Self-injury is thought to release beta-endorphins that dampen pain, and in people with diminished or absent verbal communication, self-injury might provide paradoxical respite from the distress experienced by being in physical pain.'

(Heslop and Lovell, 2013, p. 10). The other aspect is the environment: it may be that the support services around the individual are not right – they may not get on with the staff or with peers, they do not understand them; they may be rejected by their family – all of which could unsettle the person and in some instances, lead to self-harm. Being alert to this acknowledges that people with intellectual disabilities are dependent on others' support, which places them in a more vulnerable position.

Self-injury for an individual can take the form of self-punishment and blaming themselves, in which they have difficulties in communicating. It can be that they may want something tangible or a reaction from someone; this gives rise to emotions such as frustration or desire, leading to self-harm. It is a means to attempt to have control in a situation in which they have no control. How people with intellectual disability hurt themselves is different from the general population: they are more likely to bang their head, bite their hands and poke their own eyes. The main treatment option is medication, which is contentious – so much so that a government campaign has been initiated to 'Stop over-medication of people with a learning disability, autism or both' (STOMP). When people with an intellectual disability were interviewed in a study about why they self-harm and what sort of support they need, the main reason given was a 'lack of control' in their lives and the most helpful aspect of their care was being listened to and the quality of the listening. While non-verbal people were not included in this survey, this is a useful insight into what people with intellectual disabilities would like and find helpful (Heslop and Macaulay, 2009).

Sinason reminds us that we all self-harm at various points in our lives; by having an extra glass of wine or eating too much, the list could go on. We can self-harm as a form of self-medication – the challenge is to understand the individual emotional pain being expressed, too often this is denied meaning with this population. The term 'challenging behaviour' in ID services today is invariably used to describe someone with difficult behaviour.

Working with the network

One of the key challenges for the therapist is that the therapeutic relationship is not *between* a simple dyad, as the therapist is working as part of the service user's network. Working with the network is a recognized key feature of disability work (Cottis and O'Driscoll, 2009). It has been compared to child psychotherapy (Cottis, 2009) in that the therapist has to consider the relationship with the child's parents as it is important to get the parents' support. In the same way, the modern disability therapist practitioner recognizes the importance of working with care staff. It can be a challenge: Symington, for example, describes his efforts to work with his patient's support network and to enlist their support for the treatment. 'The staff were very willing to help. But to communicate what I had learned in a therapeutic encounter, through rational explanations, was only minimally successful.' (Symington, 1981, p. 192). Staff on whom we rely to bring the service user to therapy, and to support them sympathetically may be poorly paid and relatively unsupported in their ancillary roles. It may bring up conflicting feelings, for example, support workers may have an ambivalent emotional experience, having both caring feelings with a wish to help and 'repair' and feelings of anger and frustration at their inability to do so. Also, resentment for the therapist too, maybe feeling that they are having an easy time being with the patient for only 50 minutes when they are with them for up 20 hours at a time.

It is important that the person's wider network supports them having therapy and provides a containing function outside the consulting room. Confidentiality is not always respected; support workers or family may ask the person questions about the sessions. For these reasons, I often see the person with a member of their support network at our first meeting, when I explain what the psychotherapy involves, that I will see them every week, at the same time in the same room and that the session will last for 50 minutes in most cases, or perhaps 30 minutes. I explain that the sessions are private and confidential but that, if there is communication outside the session, I will always tell the service user. This is a difficult balancing act, as the network will have their own needs and expectations of the person in their care.

I am writing this in January 2021 and despite changes in social policy and government legislation, there is an obligation on the mainstream health services to find ways to adapt their services to engage people with an intellectual disability. And yet, I suspect that most psychotherapists and therapeutic organizations would flatly refuse Ms A as 'not suitable' and signpost her back to the local disabilities services. This might well be the right response. Clearly, not everybody who is non-verbal and has a moderate intellectual disability is suitable for a talking treatment. But, too often, this group gets excluded, even though, since the 1990s, there has been a growing body of psychoanalytic therapeutic literature (Sinason, 1992, Cottis, 2008, Corbett, 2019) that reports positive outcomes from such work (Shepherd and Beail, 2017).

Working with people who have intellectual disabilities requires the same fundamental skills and values as working with any other population:
- a non-judgmental attitude
- a non-directive approach
- staying open to the description of a variety of experiences
- paying attention to verbal and non-verbal information
- awareness of transference and countertransference phenomena.

All of these, I believe, are crucial. I have always found input from speech and language therapists to explain some of the communications issues helpful. I also allow time for an extended assessment over several sessions. However, the critical element is developing a relationship. This may be the first time the person has been invited to think for themselves and take responsibility for their own thoughts and feelings. The therapeutic framework in these circumstances presents a unique situation, because of the nature of learning disability and the setting. Psychotherapy can be experienced as threatening to the individual and their network, upsetting their 'equilibrium'. Working with family members can also be a challenging component. In the first meeting, I have found myself overwhelmed by relatives' psychological needs and sometimes by their difficulties in listening; the challenge of having a reciprocal conversation can seem beyond us at this point. I'm aware that the way the families present themselves may be the result of years of battling to get services and they may have anxiety about not being taken seriously. They can have important insights into how the person communicates, particularly if they are non-verbal. Here is a good example by a mother of a person who is non-verbal, 'I think it because she can't communicate and she understands so much, well a lot, but she can't communicate back. You can't understand her signings … it's like if she wants crisps or ice cream. You have to go through everything, and it gets her worked up, and in the end, she'll get you up and show you what she wants, or she'll get up and start hitting herself because she's thinking, "Are you stupid?" This is what she must be thinking, "Can you not understand me?"' (Heslop and Macaulay, 2009, p. 87).

Therapeutic challenges

All of these aspects are part of the therapeutic challenges to be aware of when working with people with ID. Certainly my mainstream psychotherapy training did not prepare me for working in this field. Parsons and Upton's (1986) survey of the experiences of Tavistock Clinic psychotherapists, found that service users presented to them had behaviours not encountered before in mainstream services. Psychotherapists are faced with behaviours that break the conventions of therapy. These included: arriving very early or late for appointments, personal questioning and inappropriate demands. Symington (1981) reported that these behaviours could dominate the psychotherapy session. He also reported his struggle to deal with the anxieties of his patient, 'Harry walked round the consulting room. I did not feel at ease just sitting down in my normal chair and watching him, so I used to stand and walk around the room as well.' (1981, p. 324). Other clinicians have reported examples. Hodges (2003) described cases of female clients displaying their vaginas or masturbating in sessions. Kahr (2017) discusses spitting and its challenges. This can also include passivity or submissive behaviours, including the handicapped smile (Sinason, 1992) to placate a more powerful other.

An example of how I worked with a service user is Ms B, who was self-harming, cutting her arms but also cutting her hair with scissors, something that caused considerable unease and confusion for her support team. Ms B started this behaviour following the death of her father and, after some discussion, it was established that she was not told about his death until just before the funeral, perhaps a period of a week or so. This is sadly not an uncommon response, as there is an anxiety around the person with an ID and their reaction to grief (O'Driscoll, 2014, 2018). I also found out that her father was a hairdresser; both of these aspects were key elements in her self-harm. I saw her for psychotherapy and we were able to focus on her putting into words her distress; she had a sense of being 'father's special girl' and of the betrayal and abandonment she felt. Maybe she was not so special after all.

Another example is of a service user who did not get the service she needed as the multidisciplinary team meeting I was part of chose a different option for her. Ms D was a new referral to our NHS service, a young woman who was displaying very concerning self-harm, cutting her arms quite severely and talking about suicide. In her network, she was causing a lot of concern. Ms D had a long history of self-harming, and had some various short-term psychological interventions at a Child and Adolescent Mental Health Services (CAMHS) team, but it was not clear how helpful this had been. She asked for 'bereavement counselling' as her mum had just died. In the team discussion around this, it was revealed that her mother had a long history of severe mental health issues. Ms D missed out on being with her mother in her last moments before she died and was refused access to attend her funeral as it was felt it would 'upset her', sadly, not an uncommon decision (O'Driscoll, 2014). During the discussion, it was revealed that she had been sexually abused by her uncle, her mum's brother. This is a classic example of being vulnerable to a complicated grief reaction. Research tells us that if the relationship is ambivalent, the greater the vulnerability to complicated grief (Dodd et al., 2008). I advised that she needed immediate long term psychoanalytic psychotherapy. However, the team decided to go in another direction and followed the advice of the nurse and the psychiatrist who felt that a mixture of medication and nursing support could contain her. This can be another challenge of being part of a service that does not always understand the attachment aspect of relationships and its vulnerability to grief. It can go for more straightforward explanations which offer simpler solutions.

In the consulting room

I like to go into the consulting room as fully briefed on the service user as I can. This is one of the benefits of working in a multidisciplinary team. I would call this 'pre-therapy work'. This would involve looking at other professional perspectives and notes. For Ms A, who was introduced at the beginning of this chapter, I was particularly interested in the speech therapist's assessment. This emphasized that Ms A's receptive language was good, which relates to the ability to understand what other people say. There are a range of communication aids including Makaton signing, (a simplified version of British Sign Language designed for people with a learning disability), but after checking, I found that Ms A did not know this. Today in services we would also have the option of 'Talking mats', or 'Life Mapping' – both are recent inventions which I did not have access to at the time.

Ms A was my first client, who was non-verbal and self-harming. She was referred for 'bereavement counselling' as there was no music therapist available. I went to meet the manager of her rather chaotic and noisy day service. The manager did not seem to have a good relationship with her. She used phrases such as 'attention-seeking' and talked about 'ignoring her bad behaviour', which I felt was clearly the wrong approach. She also wondered about increasing her medication. I was unimpressed, to say the least. Levitas and Hurley (2007) studied how support staff use medication in these situations. They discuss countertransference as a factor in the over-medication of people with intellectual disabilities, suggesting that support workers are often driven to administer PRN ('as needed') medication by their own anxieties and fear, rather than in response to any medical need in the service user. I put forward the case for individual psychotherapy and, luckily, there was an NHS consulting room available near to the service that we could use. I was concerned that the manager's scepticism might hinder the sessions and, at times, it did, as the service staff not infrequently 'forgot about sessions' and Ms A missed several.

Most people who have intellectual disabilities do not refer themselves for treatment. In the first session, I need to check if they are consenting. I explain that I know a bit about them, often from their written referral. It can be a delicate balance to gauge if they do want to attend the sessions, but one which I assess during our time together. I do not focus on the self-harm 'symptoms' as such; sometimes families or services would like it that I, 'sort out the symptoms', but I take on a holistic approach of the individual. The other key challenging aspect is the lack of personal history; I had asked the staff to talk to Ms A's sister about her childhood. I did receive a little information, but it was not very useful. This can make it very difficult to work with people with an intellectual disability, as well as the lack of staff curiosity about a person.

I remember being struck by Ms A's entry into the room. She was very tentative, like she was in trouble, or had been sent to see the headteacher. She shuffled in; it felt she believed that there was no way I would be interested and concerned about her. Ms A had an ever-present smile and an understandable anxiety, which I always address in the first instance; I pointed at myself and said, 'You don't know me, you never met me?' I felt she understood, and I told Ms A that the staff were concerned about her after her mother's death. Immediately, she stopped smiling. I commented upon this and talked about how people thought that maybe, by coming and seeing me, I might be able to help? I spoke to her about how we would be meeting in the same room to think about how she was getting on with all these changes. Gesturing to my head, I also spoke of how I was interested in what was going on in her head. Initially, I limited the sessions to 30 minutes, rather than the traditional 50 minutes. I suggested we met for five sessions and then review the therapy to see if she was happy to carry on. I remember feeling curious about working with her but also very anxious. 'When a client communication is impaired the therapist anxiety is heightened: it leaves the therapeutic dyad exposed, bereft of the protective cover of language which, as well as being a means of exchange and interaction, also offers defensive options' (Wilson, 2002, p. 82).

There is a long history of the infantilization of people with intellectual disability; Trent (1994) wrote how they went from being seen as a 'menace' at the turn of the century to being viewed as 'perpetual children' and an 'object of pity' from the 1940s. Today infantilization can take the form of being treated as a child, maybe by denying the person's sexuality, for example. When working with Ms A I initially found myself asking a lot of simple closed questions, to which Ms A 'replied' with nods or shakes of her head. I did this via a family history exercise, drawing a picture of a house, asking who lived there, i.e. her mum and dad as well as the people who visited, like her sister. I got a sense of what she could understand, to gauge if we could build a relationship, and most of all to understand her current predicament. She had lived in the same house with her parents all her life. This meant I was dealing with multiple losses. This is one of the aspects which make people with an ID vulnerable to grief, as they are dealing with a number of losses that can overwhelm the person (O'Driscoll, 2014, 2018). To help me discuss her grief, I used some materials from Books Beyond Words, a publisher specializing in texts for people with intellectual disability who find pictures easier to understand. The two books on grief I used were *When Mum Died*, about the process and effects of a parent dying, and *When Somebody Dies* on how counselling works (Hollins and Sireling, 2004, Hollins, Dowling and Blackman, 2003).

As mentioned previously, there is evidence that people with intellectual disability are more vulnerable to trauma from bereavement and are less able than the general population to process a normal grief reaction (O'Driscoll, 2014, 2018). This certainly seemed to be the case with Ms A. I also wondered if the grief was behind her self-harm? These books were useful in helping me to get behind Ms A's ever-present 'handicapped smile', which I felt she was using because she wanted to show her support services that she was 'OK and happy'. For this reason I gave her an opportunity to say that I was wrong: for example, I knew her sister did not live at home but I asked Ms A if her sister lived at home with her. She clearly said no. Then on a piece of paper I first wrote Ms A's town, asking if her sister lived there and again she said no. I then wrote her sister's home town, to which she smiled. I used other visual methods: for example, I talked to her about her current stress being 'this much', standing up and pointing up to the ceiling, whereas her stress was normally 'this much', sitting down and pointing to the table leg. She understood and nodded vigorously.

Over the course of these early sessions, I felt we were able to develop a relationship, which is the key element in a therapeutic encounter like this. This meant I could move on to discuss more painful aspects of her life. At first, Ms A struggled with some of my suggestions that, while she could acknowledge that she was sad, she was also very angry, but she did not respond to me. I did feel she was angry, and I was getting reports of her self-harming, often superficial cuts to her arms. The day centre would sometimes send notes of incidents or areas of concerns and if this happened, I would always read these out in front of her. This was often uncomfortable for her but I returned to this, and it was a few times before she would acknowledge it.

A hugely significant moment in the psychotherapy came when she turned up very late one week due to a traffic accident. Ms A was very flustered. Unfortunately, I could only see her for a short time which made her very unhappy and she started hitting herself. I spoke to her about how she was looking forward to seeing me and having her psychotherapy session, yet now I was sending her away, and she did not understand. I commented that she was cross with me and Ms A seemed to acknowledge this. I gave an extra few minutes outside the normal session time. This moment became something that I could reflect back to Ms A; by pointing at her and showing how she scratched her arms when she was angry with me I then pointed back to myself. I was showing her that the anger she felt in that moment was directed to and for me. It felt like a breakthrough moment. I was confident of this in part due to my heightened countertransference, an important feature of work with people who are non-verbal; I had this sense after working with her for a time that I was tuning into her. I was on her wavelength. But as with any therapeutic relationship, it was a bumpy ride; at times, I was not always clear if she understood me. I was anxious that I might be using too many words. I was very curious about how Ms A was getting on in her new residential setup, but it was difficult to get a clear picture here. I drew a map first with her family home and the various local amenities (via Google maps) and how she had to say goodbye to them, like the local park and shop. The shop seemed a big loss for her, which surprised me at the time. This did not work so well with her residential service; Ms A did not have much curiosity about the local area. I suspect she didn't get the opportunity to go out as much. But I also spoke about the challenges of settling in, how strange was it for her. It was not like her family home. We went back and forth with this and Ms A was able to tell me that she liked the food and having her own room. This 'simple' discussion took several sessions.

It is important that disability therapists do not flinch from the pain of disability but work with it as a part of a person's identity that affects how they relate to themselves and others. Over the course of the sessions, I tried to speak very plainly and explain what she was going through and my formulation of her situation. This was about her being 'different to others' and how that made people treat her; how upsetting this was for her at times, and that sometimes this made her do bad things to herself as her angry feelings had nowhere else to go. Her relationship with her sister was crucial here as it was clear that Ms A did not see her as much as she wanted to, and I wondered about her sister's ambivalence. We did find a way to acknowledge that this was also a big loss for her. This is a common experience for adults with an ID, a struggle to keep contact with those they care most about.

Alan Corbett, in his case study of his non-verbal patient 'Barry', who had been sexually abused, wrote of 'his struggle to bear the dead weight of Barry's silences and the exhaustion of trying to spark into life a brain that was slow and unwieldy.' (Corbett, 2019, p. 39/40). Corbett felt the key for him with Barry was his supervision with Valerie Sinason and her encouragement to explore his countertransference. While I did feel the same weight as Corbett, I certainly did at moments feel anxious, uncertain and confused. It took me some time to feel confident in exploring my countertransference rather than feeling it reflected my internal state as a novice therapist. I had many moments of boredom and maybe this is not working? This is not proper therapy. Why I am bothering? I began to notice little things at first; she started shaking her arm when she was angry. This helped me and gave me some thinking space. One time she banged her head and I felt sad, so I spoke to her about how she had been trying to bang out her bad thoughts as they were hurting. When she was late, I felt angry, and I knew she was attacking me by hurting herself in front of me. My supervision helped me and encouraged me to explore this more, particularly my hatred. 'Close encounters with disability provoke multi-layered unconscious responses. To be a psychotherapist working intensively with a disability involves the processing of hatred. This is necessary to love those parts of our patients that induce hope in us, and bring pockets of insight and attunement that oil the wheels of the therapy.' (Cottis, 2019, p. 37). After a time, I felt more relaxed, even when one week, she never spoke in the session and, after various attempts to put into words what she was feeling, I felt all she wanted was for me just to sit with her in silence. After this, I noticed that she was smiling less, seemed more serious. I felt she was more in touch with a realistic aspect of herself. I got reports from the day centre that she was more settled, however I understood that she did 'flare up' on occasions.

Despite the loss of her home and her family, Ms A settled in at her new home. I think she enjoyed a bit of freedom there, more than when she had lived with her family. She had a good and attentive key worker in the home. The keyworker was curious about the sessions but was respectful, and I encouraged her in her work with Ms A. Support staff can develop and encourage their relationships. Still, there was a fear from the keyworker about saying the right thing, but I felt this was another significant moment, to transition my support to the keyworker.

Looking back now, I wonder if I should have carried on seeing her. Over time, her self-harm decreased, and she became increasingly comfortable in her residential service. There were fewer incidents and I noticed that she became more curious about her surroundings. At the time there was a consensus from her support network that I had 'done my bit' and she needed to be left to 'get on with her new life'. I saw her for about eight months after we agreed to carry on after reviewing at five sessions, having twenty-nine sessions in total. I now think I should have insisted that I saw her for at least a year, which I try to do in most of my other disability therapy work. This was a reflection of my status as a novice therapist, still not having found my voice as a 'disability therapist'. Today I might also have tried increasing the length of sessions to 50 minutes. I wonder if I was protecting myself from the uncomfortable feelings that the silences brought up as, initially, I felt a pressure to 'think of something with which to engage Ms A', although over time this decreased. Writing about these sessions now many years later, I have a clear memory of her and them, which I don't for some of the other people I have seen. It was clearly a formative clinical experience for me. It is also worth noting that I still do not get many referrals of non-verbal service users.

Conclusions

Today, I believe we have moved a long way from asking if people with intellectual disabilities can benefit from psychotherapy. It is now established that the therapist needs to modify the psychoanalytic technique when working with this client group (Sinason, 1992). This means that the therapist needs to work with greater flexibility and willingness to engage with the wider systems. Historically, a few practitioners have worked with people with intellectual disabilities, and I have written elsewhere about this early history, which up until 1980 was characterized by 'moments of curiosity', rather than a sustained, cumulative body of research. The organization I currently chair, the Institute of Psychotherapy and Disability (https://instpd.org.uk), surveyed all adult psychotherapy and counselling training organizations back in 2010 and found only one that worked with people with intellectual disabilities, the John Bowlby Centre (https://thebowlbycentre.org.uk). Most did not even reply. How seriously this is taken is reflected in the IAPT (Improving Access to Psychological Therapies) website, where a planned page on working with people with intellectual disability was still blank in April 2019. Again we must look to the work of Valerie Sinason, for illumination on this and her quote 'the widespread wish for medical science to eradicate intellectual disability means that those born and living "with it" are not emotionally welcome nor included.' While Corbett has written strongly about the 'profoundly low levels of self-esteem, agency and psychic integrity felt by people with intellectual disability [that] stem more from all that is projected into them from birth (and beyond) than from the actual fact of their low IQ' (Corbett, 2014, p. 8).

People with ID who self-injure have the same need for emotional support as people without ID who self-harm. By failing to realize this we will forever be regarding self-injury in people with ID as a complex problem that requires containment rather than psychological care. I also think that supervision of disability psychotherapy needs to include a space for thinking about ways of working with the non-verbal. Getting comfortable in an endlessly silent room, enduring the uncertainties, doubts and mysteries that the silence only make greater, is the therapist's task of 'negative capability' (Keats, 1817). Admittedly, it is not an easy one. The lack of spoken communication can be stressful. The time it takes to unravel and discover the most simple information can be challenging. In my view, we as a profession need to find a way to use our own spaces, our supervision and training, to discuss our fears and anxieties in order to be of real service to this vulnerable and richly deserving group.

CHAPTER 4

Patients who smell: olfactory communication and the mephitic other

Gabrielle Brown

This chapter explores ways of thinking about the meaning of smell and odour in psychotherapeutic interventions with individuals who neglect or resist current conventions of personal hygiene. Psychoanalytic thought has largely eschewed the challenge of addressing dirt and body odour. By contrast, social history and political theory have a long-standing fascination with the 'unwashed' – the non-compliant poor – (Corbin, 1982/1986; Stallybrass and White, 1986; Cockayne, 2007; Cox et al., 2011; Jenner, 2000, 2011 inter alia) and with tracing the designation of excluded social groups as dirty and pungent. The formation of what I term a 'social countertransference', which confers psychological meaning upon communication via odour, is therefore relatively under-theorized. The human sense of smell is the most subjective and least verifiable of the senses (Cobb, 2020), the most subject to both imaginative construction and prejudice. In the post-industrial and more sanitary contemporary environment, when we say that someone 'smells', we actually mean that they smell of themselves. The 'dirt' we wash from ourselves no longer comes from muddy streets but rather comes from *within* the body and is produced by the body itself: sweat, urine, faeces, menstrual products, sebum and so on (Lagerspetz, 2018). It is the very personal nature of the communication, in the context of a very emphatic psychosocial response, that makes it an important area for consideration.

The issue of smell is also fascinating because in twenty-first-century Western culture, our response to those smells considered 'bad' has a marked and frank immediacy. Without a second thought, the malodorous individual is considered beyond the pale – responses to smells considered 'bad' take the quality of instinctive reaction to threat and do not raise debate, reflection or sympathy. Liberal discourses on social exclusion that question why any member of society should ever be excluded stall on the issue of 'offensive' odour. It is, for instance, impossible to conceive of public policies of non-discrimination and inclusiveness towards those who neglect personal hygiene. And while many liberal societies value not *taking offence* as highly as *not giving offence*, a zero-tolerance towards personal odour remains the norm. By the same token, both historically and in the current era, the designation of individuals and groups as 'dirty' and 'smelly' both legitimizes invisible boundaries to a society's hospitality and distribution of resources and organizes stigma.

In our age of scientific rationalism, the startled response to the malodorous is almost completely irrational. While evolutionary biology notes that 'disgust' is registered by a cerebrally primitive part of the brain's insula, the majority of responses carried over from earlier 'primitive' life forms are culturally modified in contemporary human societies (Miller, 2004). Twenty-first-century scientific knowledge directs fear away from odour as the primary source of disease and harm, to toxins and pollutants that the human senses cannot detect. In the time of the Covid-19 pandemic, detection of any odour is personally preferable to none, as anosia, loss of sense of smell, is a disease symptom and social distancing has reduced the olfactory richness of lived experience. Even before Covid, odourless dangers of radiation, air pollution and chemical residues from food production, radically restructured conceptions of the relationship between dirt and harm. Dirt's danger no longer simply equates to harbouring micro-organisms such as bacteria, because 'good bacteria' – for instance, in the human gut biome – along with the global problems of the overuse of antibiotics, encourage a more discriminating view (Spector, 2015). But current medical materialism has in no way moderated our emphatic reaction to the odorous, nor our increasing emphasis on the importance of washing and de-odourizing the body to produce a narrow olfactory palette of flowers and fruit for the body and mint for the breath. The linguistic trace of our preoccupation with being 'odourless' is found in the way the term 'hygiene' – etymologically the 'art of health' or more widely 'well being' – has contracted in modern usage to denote only cleanliness (Oxford Dictionaries, 2018b). Although our 'personal hygiene' routines are in fact historically recent, they are considered innate and instinctive to human nature, marshalled by fear of being shamed by our physiological functions and their odours (Mollon, 1993, 2005). In the anthropocene, the era of human impact on the Earth's environment, bathing daily in heated water damages the planet's climate and its oceans. Thus presenting as 'nice and clean' may come to figure, in retrospect, as more perversely narcissistic and antisocial than its opposite. But there are, I will argue, deep cultural and unconscious underpinnings preventing us from uncoupling the association between smelling 'fresh' on the one hand and care for the body and the lived environment on the other.

Understanding issues of smell conceptually in psychoanalytic terms tends to be avoided in the same way as the 'smelly' person is avoided physically. Clinicians agonize about whether and when to mention evident smell to the patient, rather than what to make of it (Anzieu, 1996 [1985]). Anzieu describes a tendency to 'counter-transferential resistance' to somatic communication, such as odour: 'thinking that the most noticeable material produced in the sessions could not have anything to do with psychoanalysis because it was neither verbalised nor had any apparent communicative value.' (Anzieu, 1996[1985], p. 200) Being 'smelly' tends to be viewed as accidental oversight, not as meaningfully communicative – the olfactory equivalent of talking to oneself in public. Psychiatric diagnosis is similarly dismissive: while both 'self-neglect' and the behavioural reverse – compulsive washing – appear within the pages of manuals (APA, 2013), only obsessional cleanliness has the status of an illness, related to a state of mind and personal history. Abstaining from washing tends to be omitted from clinical formulation and is seen rather as direct laziness or an antisocial stance.

Psychoanalytic ideas of 'symptoms', which themselves reflect complex unconscious internal states, problematize the designation of self-neglect as a deliberate antisocial act from which individuals can easily abstain, if they so wish. Rather, an intrapsychic view suggests that failures of 'selfcare' stem from a disturbed and traumatized relationship between the individual and his or her body, first and foremost. From a developmental perspective, a tendency to communicate distress through the body – 'somatically' – relates to pre-verbal communication between the baby and those who nurture him or her (see Anzieu, 1996 [1985]; Sidoli, 1996; Segal, 1997; Hilty, this volume). Enduring habits of primarily somatic communication may result from experiences of failures in early nurturing. The failure of 'self-care' in adult life develops in individuals who lacked thoughtful understanding and responses from the minds of others at the formative start of their lives, even if they received enough physical care to survive.

In this chapter, I will seek to bring concepts from our rich psychoanalytic canon to bear on this relatively neglected 'symptom' of dirt and smell. Psychoanalysis enables a variety of perspectives on the individual meaning of the symptom and also the significance of our response – individual and psychosocial – to it. I will suggest that malodorousness is a communication that both demonstrates and obscures sites of internal psychic pain. I will set psychoanalytic exploration alongside the lively sociological and historical literature that gives a psychosocial hinterland to our current assumptions about the meaning of an apparently antisocial self-presentation. As psychotherapists, our responses to the unwashed patient in particular, and to communication with or via the body in general, are embedded in current social attitudes. Our therapeutic countertransference is readily coloured by a 'social countertransference' rooted in historically determined assumptions about the meaning of 'poor hygiene' and, more generally, the unconscious use of the body in the communication of mental states. Therefore the 'smelly' patient rarely evokes therapeutic curiosity and formulation nor, at the level of affective response, pity or concern.

I will draw on social anthropologist Mary Douglas' classic work *Purity and Danger* (1966) to see our response to 'invasive' odours as resonant with deeper fears about the demands of others upon our material and emotional resources. The socially excluded, homeless, destitute and mentally ill in our midst are individuals whose distress and discomfort are not well contained by the given structuring opposites in society – private/public, asylum/community, individual/communal, secret/ostentatious, indoors/outside and so on. Odours cross a somatic boundary unavoidably. While we can avert our gaze from what we would rather not see, we are helpless and passive recipients of odours. The evocative communication via the sense of smell reminds us of the permeability between our mind and the minds of others and the psychic processes that may occur around the boundary between self and other. Intolerance of the smells of others, more even than others' noise, stimulates our narcissistic difficulty with human relatedness and interdependence that Bion termed the 'problem of groupishness' (Bion, 1961, p. 131).

The conceptual and historical territories

> Generically, of course, West Indians were not dirty. However we were seen, metaphorically, to be *'like dirt'*, in Mary Douglas's more profound sense of 'matter out of place'.
> *Familiar Stranger: A Life Between Two Islands*, by S. Hall p. 189

Dirt and disorder

Mary Douglas (1966) provides a powerful conceptual framework for the exploration of social meanings of 'being dirty' and odorous. In *Purity and Danger*, she traces the needs of human societies to delineate categories and systems of 'clean' and 'unclean'. These categories provide orientation that is both ontological and constitutive of general social systems and relations: 'Reflection on dirt involves reflection on the relation of order to disorder, being to non-being, form to formlessness, life to death.' (Douglas, 1966, p. 5). Douglas contends that the border or threshold between structural opposites – for instance between life/death, individual/communal, us/them – forms sites of social anxiety and of responses to that anxiety. Social systems manage deeper existential anxiety by defining and controlling manifest categories, such as dirty/clean: dirt 'implies two conditions: a set of ordered relations and a contravention of that order. Dirt, then, is never a unique, isolated event. *Where there is dirt there is system*.' (Douglas, 1966, p. 35; emphasis added).

One consequence of the use of symbolic conventions to manage deeper social and existential anxieties is that we systematize an illogical but deep horror of anything that challenges those conventions (Menninghaus, 2003). 'Our idea of dirt is compounded of two things: care for hygiene and respect for conventions.' (Douglas, 1966, p. 7).

The return of the repressed

In considering the nature of the human senses, Freud's phylogenic view was typically post-Enlightenment, with sight and hearing privileged over the 'animal' senses of touch and smell (Freud, 1930). In Freud's narrative of human evolution, the human acquisition of upright gait removed the nose from closeness to the genitals and excretory organs of other members of the species (Freud, 1930; Mollon, 2005). I will return to some other consequences of phylogenic and ultimately social Darwinist views of the evolution of the species in the next section, in the construction and consequences of distinctions between human 'races'.

Freud suggested that only in 'perversions' is the human sense of smell still dominant as 'perversions' 'regularly have an animal character' (Freud, 1985 [1897], p. 223), with fetishism particularly related to smell (Freud, 1905, p. 155 note). 'Civilized' society therefore aims to be free from odour and the need to attend to its significance in order to 'bind', repress or sublimate the animal and sexual instincts that the sense of smell may stimulate. But the subliminal nature of reception of odour (Cobb, 2020), and its invisible, drifting character, evokes the permeability of the barrier between our unconscious and conscious mind and thereby the return of the repressed. The reception of both good and bad smells gives a vista of failures of repression, disavowal and negation that may be sexually inviting or uncannily frightening. The precariousness of repression of the pungent and sexual is often itself a site of excitement: many English euphemisms for the sexual refer to dirt (e.g. smutty, rank, filthy), while the popular imagination still relishes Napoleon's supposed request to Josephine not to bathe – '*ne te lave pas, je reviens*'. By the same token, refusing 'cleanliness' can carry valuable countercultural cachet, as in Joan Baez's description of Bob Dylan as: 'already a legend/*The unwashed phenomenon*, the original vagabond …' (Joan Baez, 'Diamonds and Rust', 1975, my emphasis).

The Mephitic Other

Historian Mark Jenner's work on smells in the Early Modern period details how the feared Other is perceived to pollute the dominant social group via attributed odour (Jenner, 2000, 2011). Thus odour's penetrative quality comes to signify risk of moral and socio-political incursion. The over-determination of our intolerant response to smells with both ontological and sociopolitical attributes has created long histories of social exclusion and genocidal scapegoating, of which I will give a few salient examples in the space available. I hope to sketch the way in which attributions of 'stench' become, in different contexts, markers of difference that is eschatological, moral and phylogenic. These social constructions give rise to pseudoscientific hierarchies in the human species that inflect contemporary patterns of social exclusion, violence and disentitlement. One consequence is the formation of assumptions that some social groups and their symptoms are more suitable for 'talking therapies' than others.

Foetor Judaicus

Jay Geller's extensive studies of the structuring and reach of early modern anti-Semitism describe how: '[N]oxious … smells recall the repulsive, feminized, and often sexualized "odor" that pervaded the popular and scientific imagination of post-emancipation Europeans: the innate stench of the Jew, the *"foetor Judaicus"*. It's a completely different aesthetic register with which to think through European anti-Semitism and German Jewish thought and culture.' (Geller, 2011, p. 35). The distinctive Jewish stench could only be removed by Christian baptism, without which it broadcast the moral turpitude of the Jews' alleged responsibility for Jesus Christ's death. Freud was well aware of the tight conceptual nexus between races considered pungent and theories of epidemic disease. He wrote to Christian author Romain Rolland, 'I of course belong to a race which in the Middle Ages was held responsible for all epidemics and which today is blamed for the disintegration of the Austrian Empire.' He then goes on to describe living with such undercurrents of trans-historical prejudice and 'illusion' (or delusion) as 'sobering' and 'not conducive to make one believe in illusions. A great part of my life's work (I am 10 years older than you) has been spent [trying to] destroy illusions of my own and those of mankind.' (Freud, 1961 [1923], p. 326).

'Olfactory racism'

Nowhere are the 'illusions' of attributed smell and dirtiness more enduring and consequential in Western culture than the creation of notions of racial and cultural difference based on skin colour. 'Olfactory racism' as Andrew Kettler terms it in his study of how phylogenic and 'scientific' racism legitimized the Atlantic slave trade, operated 'regardless of material odors [sic] or patterns of hygiene' (Kettler, 2020, p. 38). In *The Smell of Slavery* Kettler describes in distressing detail how 'potent European cultural knowledge altered the biological function of the five senses to create an olfactory consciousness made to sense the other as foul.' (Kettler, 2020, p 38). The association of black skin with 'foulness' is inflected through notions that some races are less 'civilized' and therefore less evolved from animal origins than others (Fryer, 1984/2018). In this construction, animals are seen as more attentive to odour than human beings. Non-white races were cast as phylogenically more 'primitive' or animal-like in the expression of emotion and in the failure of repression of instinctual drives (Hall, 2018, pp. 188–9). In the use of the term 'primitive', we can trace the constant slippage between the ontogenic use meaning 'of infancy', found in psychoanalytic discourse and the phylogenic association with lesser evolutionary development. This slippage renders some races 'primitive' – more instinctual, less capable of rational thought, even childlike: therefore, much less capable of understanding the importance of cleanliness and hygiene and of attending to it. Thus racialized constructions of difference interpenetrate perceptions of cultural difference, 'converting cultural differences into racial categories, and physical markers into civilizational ones, turns out to be a key mechanism in the discourse of difference' (Hall, 2018, p. 189). Hall's contention that 'race' is an empty or 'floating' signifier (equivalent to Freud's 'illusion' above) allows those considered 'odourous' or 'foul' to be seen as engaged in a process of undermining civilized communication. A failure to abstain from communicating via the body, a failure to be properly 'clean', takes human evolution down a notch, forcing out the rational with the olfactory. We can see the trace of these discriminatory attitudes in therapeutic assumptions that, unlike other symptoms, there is nothing to *say* about odour. As if the patient had slipped beyond the realm of verbal communication into a more 'primitive' animal-like world that is beyond psychoanalytic reach.

The 'great unwashed'

> As the bourgeoisie produced new forms of regulation and prohibition governing their own bodies, they wrote ever more loquaciously of the body of the other – the city's 'scum'.
> *The Politics and Poetics of Transgression*
> P. Stallybrass and A. White (1986, p. 126)

Contemporary reactions to the malodorous also bear the historical trace of deep concerns about urban social relations in terms of illness, mortality, morality and class conflict. Until the late nineteenth century, the lethal effect of bad smells was considered a scientific fact (Bourke, 2005; Hempel, 2006; Cox et al., 2011, Naphy and Roberts, 1997). Putrid smelling air – 'miasma' – was seen as both the source of fatal diseases such as cholera and smallpox and the means of their epidemic transmission: Smells that we might consider as unpleasant could be as 'fatal as mustard gas.' (Jenner, 2000, p. 4). In London, for instance, Victorian miasmists saw deadly odours emanating from the slums of the East End's poor, whose fetid living conditions were attributed to fecklessness, vice and eugenic degeneration (Cox et al., 2011). Edwin Chadwick (1842, p. 124), wrote of the 'unutterable horrors' of the city, where there were no 'architectural barriers or protections of decency and propriety'. The great sanitary reformers of the nineteenth-century European city – Bazalgette and Chadwick in London and Haussman in Paris – were all miasmists, often vehemently opposed to the newly emerging 'germ theory' of disease (Hempel, 2006). Anxiety about disease resonated with wider concerns about sedition in the 'great unwashed', the newly formed, restless, urban working class. Haussman's designs for wide Parisian boulevards in the post-revolutionary Paris of the 1850s gave the cavalry better access to working class areas, while at the same time opening the city to light and air to dispel miasma. Smell and dirt continue very concretely to signal potential damage to the 'socially included' members of society from the socially marginalized, especially the homeless. For instance, many metropolitan councils sluice down their pavements at night, even during heavy rain, to displace the 'human grime' sleeping there.

Applying psychoanalysis: individuals

It is worth noting the paradigm shifts in our conceptions of various sorts of boundaries and their crossing that started in the nineteenth century and perhaps frame current assumptions. These shifts include the transition from a 'bad air' or *miasma* theory of disease to a germ theory – a move from a notion of the body poisoned from without to one of it attacked by germs from within. Arguably, the shift to germ theory and beyond overlaps with psychoanalysis's discovery of the unconscious mind and the mysterious emanations from unacknowledged parts of the psyche into conscious thought and action along with involuntary projection of thoughts, feelings and attributes into the minds of others. Unconscious thoughts and feelings are not in essence bounded by the morality or social contract of conscious life. Communication by odour has resonance with the universal difficulties of our psychic functioning – difficulties containing our thoughts and feelings within our own minds, the unbidden return of the repressed and the potential suffocating claustrophobia of our own internal space, which Melanie Klein saw as the roots of our existential loneliness (Klein, 1993 [1963]).

A bodily ego

Freud's postulation that the 'ego is first and foremost a bodily ego' (1923, p. 26) has enabled psychoanalysis to make sporadic comment on the meaning of smell or odour as a symptom or form of communication (e.g. Brill, 1932; Friedman, 1959; Peto, 1973; Anzieu, 1996 [1985]; Segal, 1997; Lemma, 2015). Freud noted that somatic expression of distress could enable care of the body to assist with healing the mind. In observing casualties from the First World War, he noted that those recovering from physical injury had a better prognosis for recovery from psychological trauma – 'shell shock' – than soldiers whose trauma had no physical representation (Freud, 1920). The notion of a link between the body and the care of the mind is salient in work with people who, most ostensibly, neglect routines for the care of the body and both harm their bodies and damage their 'prospects'. Additionally, Freud and his followers suggest a model of the mind and its relation to the external world that is similar to a body and its physical boundaries. The physical processes of eating, ingesting, digesting, voiding and spitting out form the models for psychological communication between the mind and external world. Psychic processes of projection, incorporation and the 'metabolism' or processing of experiences have their physical counterparts. This is more than a relationship of analogy; rather, the body, Freud suggests, may actually 'speak' for and about the mind (Breuer and Freud, 1895, p. 148). In mysterious nineteenth-century physical afflictions of hysteria, he found that the body 'join[s] the conversation' (Breuer and Freud, 1895, p. 296).

Dimensions of neglect

The neglected, rejected, unwashed body becomes noticeable or 'loquacious' through the smell it produces. We may assume there to be repetitive patterns of unconscious self-expression in the inability to keep bad smells and bad experiences within private and secret domains of the body, the family and the home. The NICE (2009, p. 68) guidelines on *'When to suspect child mistreatment'* underline dirt and smell as important messages of distress that children often cannot articulate verbally. Furthermore, children who actively create smell by incontinence or smearing faeces may be communicating private experiences of sexual abuse and trauma.

A patient, remembering his childhood in a violent family home, describes a sense of communicating confusion and helplessness through repeated incontinence:

> That's me, the child in the corner, mumbling, pissing, shitting myself. And no one knows why. No one's asking, and I don't know, but I keep on doing it, so they leave me to it. I mean, what would you do with a kid like that?

This patient describes patterns of non-comprehension, in his own mind and those of the adults around him, towards the noticeable symptoms of his distress. Significantly, he is also commenting on the transference in therapy, where little effort is made by the homelessness system's tolerant psychotherapist to think through the specificity of his distress, thus repeating the 'seen but not heard' agony of his childhood, that I will discuss more generally below.

Dimensions of abuse

> Many men and women spend their lives wondering whether to find a solution by suicide, that is sending the body to death which has already happened to the psyche.
> 'Fear of Breakdown' *International Review of Psycho-Analysis*,
> 1, D. W. Winnicott (1974, p. 106)

The individual's failure to care for his or her adult body repeats scenarios of early neglect or abuse that enduringly dominate the internal psychic landscape. On one level, odour speaks of the avoidance of further impingement or intrusion, functioning to keep others at a distance. Sidoli (1996, p. 176) comments on the protective and defensive function of odour in her work with a child patient who 'used his farts to create a container for his infant self ... Like a skunk, he both protected himself and attacked his enemies with a barrier of poisonous smell.' However, in adult work, we are perhaps too ready to interpret more passive odorous states – being unwashed rather than more actively farting or sweating, for example – as simply hostility or withdrawal. In discussing different lines of thought in relation to the following fictionalized case example, I hope to offer some ways of thinking about why we are more likely to feel alarmed or even assaulted by 'bad smells' in the consulting room than by the content of verbal communication and fantasies.

> Tom lives in a hostel for homeless men with chronic mental health problems. At times he drinks heavily. In his many years in the hostel, Tom has never washed, and sleeps fully clothed, usually in an armchair not the bed. Hostel staff and the wider care system have come to accept his idiosyncratic 'habits' with diminishing hopes of further social integration. However, despite his reputation as 'withdrawn' and uncommunicative, he seeks out psychotherapy when it is made available.

As Lemma (2010, p. 33) comments in her study of body modification in adult life, 'the body never ceases to signal the relationship with the mother'. If Tom's inability to wash himself is seen as 'self-neglect', this repeats the profound neglect that enabled abusive sexual intrusion throughout his childhood. There is no comfort or warmth to be gained from his current relationship with his body – it is a site of profound distrust. In the consulting room, I want to sit further away from him. This alerts us to the achingly paradoxical dilemma of his childhood – where distance meant neglect, closeness, abuse.

Sexual abuse itself leaves a sense of 'betrayal by the body', a feeling that the body has colluded with the abuser in enduringly torturing the mind (Gardner, 1999, p. 140). Indeed Tom treats his body as an alien betrayer and eschews any private relationship with it – he never sees himself naked because he never gets undressed. The relationship between his body and mind is hostile as well as wary. His body is used, instrumentally, as a 'thing', a means to bring alcohol to his brain, to numb and comfort his mind. Through alcoholism and the attendant life-shortening perils of homelessness, he enacts a psychosomatic vengeance on the treacherous body. As I will describe, mind and body have been at odds from the start. Just as his mind is overwhelmed by his early traumas, so over time his body is broken by his alcoholic use of it. In this context, there is an unconscious identification with the abuser's contempt for the integrity of the child's body; an identification re-enacted in self-neglect and broadcast through odour.

It is always easier to 'hear' about endured mental and physical torture than to reconstruct original suffering from the way in which the patient has come to treat others or themselves. Tom's somatic communication places us at the scene of the crimes he has endured, by placing us in contact with the minds of both perpetrator and victim, who remain unbearably in conflict within his internal world. For instance, Tom's 'social death' – the socially taboo nature of his malodourous presentation – speaks of a deeper suicidal state and a more chronic identification with the mind of the abuser. At the start of my work with Tom, I can sense this identification in the maternal transference – in the suffocating air of the consulting room, we are both respectively soiled and sullied – a damaged mother and child. The abuser's wish to deprive a neglectful or unprotective mother of a healthy child, through sexual abuse, is internalized by the child as chronically suicidal self-neglect: '[in suicidal fantasy] the [adult] child wants to rob the parents of their greatest and most precious possession, his own life ... the punishment the child imposes upon himself is simultaneously punishment he imposes on the instigators of his sufferings' (Stekel, 1967 [1910], p. 87).

For the therapist, it may be less the pungent odour that is unbearable than the sense of unthinkable conflicts and split-identifications that are still so active in the mind of the adult patient. It is as if we can smell the actively destructive, hostile and 'perpetrator' parts of the psyche as well as the dying psyche of the child. And, unlike our response to verbal communication, it is more difficult to activate intellectualized defences against the impact of the patient's olfactory communication. More generally, many of us have a technical insecurity and impoverished vocabulary for speaking about bodily communication in the consulting room.

'Failure of indwelling'

Winnicott helpfully challenges the assumption that a coherent relationship between the mind and the body is an innate human characteristic. Rather he contends that 'psychosomatic collusion' (Winnicott, 1974, p. 103) is a developmental achievement, a capacity for 'indwelling' facilitated by devoted care for the baby, '[t]he whole routine of care through the day and night' (Winnicott, 1990 [1960], p. 48).

Anzieu (1996 [1985]) follows Winnicott's ideas in suggesting the existence of an early 'Skin Ego' in which the sense of self is constituted by the body's containing surface, rather than a sense of an internal core. An 'olfactory wrapping' or 'olfactory envelope' houses the early ego. This container is constituted by the smell of baby, 'mother' and the intuitive processes between them that enable feeding and communication (Anzieu, 1996 [1985], p. 210). We can think of Tom's early experience as a failure of a protective container and for much of his homeless adult life he has avoided living inside a house, with its symbolic resonance with maternal space (Campbell, 2019). He represents people whose early life has left them 'frightened out of their skin', and who subsequently refuse to get back into it, continuing to live as if outside the body. As he never gets undressed, he lives 'inside-out': aspects of the self deemed most intimate – how we all smell close up – are kept on the outside.

The early evolving mind–body relationship is damaged by interruptions in care, which are experienced as somatic traumas, precognitive 'primitive agonies' that enduringly haunt the individual (Winnicott, 1974). Terrors of falling apart, falling through space, of the mind having no 'say' over the body (as in fantasies of paralysis or violation) continue to lurk at the back of the mind. Winnicott's (1974, p. 105) list of these 'primitive agonies' is not exhaustive – he ends it with 'And so on'. In terms both of odour itself and its removal through washing, I would suggest that terrors of loss of a coherent state through dissolving, evaporating, leaking and leaching are salient. Tom's liminal but odorous social existence can be understood as demonstrative of his deep sense being internally precarious and incoherent, which is also expressed in his ghostlike, unseen or overlooked existence as a homeless man in the urban environment.

The interpersonal context

Loneliness and having much 'in common'

If we think of the ego as a bodily ego, then our sense of smell allows others to affect us with their communication, whether inviting, hostile or aversive. As I have suggested, smell provides a reminder of the permeability of our emotional selves to the experiences of others and, by the same token, others' receptiveness to thoughts and feelings we direct towards them. From psychoanalysis' early roots in hypnotism and mesmerism stem ideas of individual minds profoundly affecting each other in ways over which there is no conscious control (Borossa, 2001). Communication by odour bears close analogy to the psychical processes of projection, introjection and projective identification. In projective identification, for example, 'we are inclined to attribute to other people – in a sense, to put into them – some of our own emotions and thoughts' (Klein, 1993 [1959], p. 252).

The origins of the word 'communicate' are in sharing or having something 'in common' – from the Latin *communis*, communal (Oxford Dictionaries, 2018a). Odour provides something in common without the use of speech, allowing us to 'get through to each other' unavoidably. Melanie Klein (1993 [1963]) suggests that the experience of reciprocal intuitive communication between minds contributes significantly to a sense of 'belonging', inclusion and friendship – 'having something in common'. However, this reciprocity of projection and introjection becomes frightening when the boundary between our minds and those of others feels too permeable and communication too involuntary. Klein and her followers consider a feeling of excessive permeability of the self to typify psychotic types of experience (Klein, 1993 [1963]; Rosenfeld, 1960).

In disturbed and psychotic states of mind, the fragmentation of the ego becomes extreme, leaving the individual with a sense of having too much 'in common' and no boundaries around a private self. He or she is unsure which thoughts and feelings are his or her own and which belong to others; 'he constantly feels himself not only to be in bits, but to be *mixed up with* other people' (Klein, 1993 [1963], p. 304; emphasis added). The desire for common understanding or being understood collapses into an urgent need to achieve distance and separation. Klein's (1993

[1963], p. 304) important insight is that the 'constant use of withdrawal' obscures the fact that the psychotic individual 'longs to be able to make relationships with people, but cannot'. This unhappy paradox is evident in the way in which strong body odour is simultaneously invasive and aversive: that is, a communication that drives away others by making them feel that they are too close.

Suffocation and dread

Following Klein's ideas of the self 'mixed up' with others, Bion (2007 [1962]) places the need for reciprocity in communication within a developmental context. He considers the baby's first communication to be an urgent demand to the (m)other to establish a mutual field of understanding in relation to intolerable states of mind. In evocative terms, he describes the baby feeling that he or she is dying. If the mother does not respond to this fear – for instance, if the infant is neglected – the baby is overwhelmed by his or her own unmodified anxiety: a 'nameless dread' (Bion, 2007 [1962], p. 116). I have suggested that, in feeling suffocated by another's odour, we experience wholesale his or her overwhelmed internal world, which is suffused and choked by inexplicable or 'unnamed' fears and anxieties (Brown, 2013). Klein suggests that feeling overwhelmed by ourselves is a universal existential state: 'complete understanding and acceptance of one's own emotions, phantasies and anxieties is not possible and this continues as an important factor in loneliness.' (Klein, 1963, p. 302).

In receiving evidence of others' suffocation in their own distress we also receive an aversive reminder of our own.

Applying psychoanalysis: social countertransference

Dirty protest: container and contained

Odour very concretely signals a difficulty in containing intimate aspects of the self, which, I suggest, are felt to be unmanageable and 'namelessly' alien. In the interpersonal or social field it is important to acknowledge that the individual may have been expected to contain and 'manage' projected desires, attitudes and feelings from others, as well as his or her own confusing emotions. Here we touch on the complex area in which those who have been neglected or abused in intimate and primary relationships come to develop the identity of offensive scapegoats in the wider world (Behr and Hearst, 2005). In this last section I will briefly suggest readings of works of Fairbairn and Freud that help us to understand the process and meaning of becoming 'offensive'.

Fairbairn (2006 [1943]) suggests that the delinquent child (which may include the child who refuses to wash, soils or behaviourally 'makes a stink') engages in a psychic process of surviving the cruelty and 'badness' of the parental system upon which he or she depends. He suggests that maltreated children become 'containers' for a perverse and malign emotional environment through a type of absorptive introjection, taking all that is rotten and corrupt in their affective milieu into themselves. By adopting the role of 'problem' in a damaging system, these children are able to imagine being surrounded by benign, blameless and nurturing objects or people: 'outer security is thus purchased at the price of inner insecurity' (Fairbairn, 2006 [1943], p. 65). In terms that resonate with Mary Douglas's structuring ontological oppositions, Fairbairn (2006 [1943], p. 66) posits that the maltreated child reinstates the moral opposites of Christian society by taking on the role of 'scapegoat': 'it is better to be a sinner in a world ruled by God than to live in a world ruled by the Devil'. The reprehensively stinking child also re-establishes moral judgement and condemnation into a system that has been experienced as amoral and unaccountable.

The melancholic object

We can also read Freud's account of the formation, persistence and meaning of 'melancholic' symptoms in adults as a psychosocial theory of response to immoral humiliation and cruelty from the world at large. In 'Mourning and Melancholia' Freud (1917) distinguishes between the process of giving up a lost object in grief and the aggrieved refusal to relinquish the abandoning or traumatizing object in melancholia. The object is taken into the melancholic's ego and the melancholic's whole demeanour then becomes a complaint and accusation against the object's damaging cruelty. The shadow of this object stunts and stultifies the ego, blocking light and air, as it were, and rendering the melancholic's internal world dank and stale. 'Feelings of shame in front of other people are lacking in the melancholic .... one might emphasise the presence in him of an almost opposite trait of insistent communicativeness which finds satisfaction in self-exposure' (Freud, 1917, p. 240). While personal odour is usually intensely shameful, melancholic symptoms speak of a different sort of psychosocial pain. Freud is arguing, importantly, that it is psychologically naive and therapeutically fruitless to see the melancholic as the sole author of his or her own woes, when the actions, omissions and projections of another are so clearly implicated in these symptoms. In relation to 'self-neglect', a neglectful object or Other is always implicated in the symptom.

In the familiar paradox of symptoms, the stinking child or 'self-neglecting' adult makes something rotten and inequitable manifest in the very process of obscuring its source within his or her emotional environment. Therefore, the effect of the Other needs to be brought to light alongside the intentions and responsibility of the melancholic him- or herself. The accused Other in the delinquent and melancholic demonstrative narrative is not always a person but can equally be a condition of being in the world – being thwarted, humiliated or reviled, situated as an outcast, or living precariously in a society whose very structure is based upon 'casting out' or 'putting people in their place' (Gilligan, 1996; Bauman, 2004; Adlam and Scanlon, 2009; Scanlon and Adlam, 2019). It follows from this perspective that politely seeking to relate to the 'person beneath the odour' in the consulting room sidesteps the moral poignancy of the patient's position and the significance of his or her history. While stinking in public continues to be perceived as grossly antisocial, personal odour must be seen as an address to moral thought in the therapist, rather than to their olfactory prejudice. Any antisocial symptom, however unconsciously produced, demands a moral archaeology of its etiology. Fairbairn helps us see that we can think of the 'offensiveness' of the malodourous as an appeal for a moral examination of the origins and meaning of their symptoms.

Conclusions

Many people who neglect personal hygiene are very 'locked in' to their own minds and overwhelmed – very lonely. In opting for therapy there is hope of finding themselves more tolerable – if a therapist can bear them, then perhaps they can come to bear themselves too. Such individuals do not want to avoid contact with the minds of others – a stereotype of the reasons for being 'smelly'. Rather they need intimate, deeply shameful parts of the internal world to be known and this is one way to understand why the patient may bring their intimate and shameful odours to their therapist. The olfactory volume of these somatic communications is often turned up too high – being smelly has a similar insistence to shouting. However, from a developmental perspective, such individuals have had little experience, in childhood or adulthood, of anyone choosing to listen, rather than simply react, to them. As the chapters in this book detail, people who communicate through or with the body have very poor access to talking therapies and the dilemmas of their internal world have only sporadically preoccupied psychoanalytic thought, despite the well-known psychological origins of their trauma.

It stands to reason that the body carries communication of those aspects of experience that are most difficult to put into words. Often the experience has been of traumatic breach of social taboos – of sexual abuse, neglect and violence in the home, discrimination, stigma, exclusion and violence in the wider world, resulting in hopeless and murderous feelings towards the self and its objects. I suggest it is no accident that the individual in turn invokes a moral compass in others and activates social condemnation and taboo in communicating the lasting psychic impact of early experiences – with being 'smelly' in public an occasion for social opprobrium *par excellence*. For therapists (and other workers), declining to be 'touched' by the painful dilemmas signalled by strong olfactory communication constitutes 'not neutrality but falseness or imperviousness' (Brenman Pick, 1985, p. 163). Psychoanalyst Irma Brenman Pick makes these remarks in a technical paper on the therapist's need to 'work through' his or her countertransference reaction to the patient's feelings and situation in order to keep 'love and concern' alive.

When individuals' smells suffuse public space, 'they' make 'us' feel claustrophobic, irrationally suffocated, intensely worried there is not enough air to go round. I have traced how our current social attitudes to the 'smelly' are steeped in historical constructions of the 'Other' as threatening Christian civilization and its moralized order via odour, neglect of cleanliness and disease. Many of these attitudes cannot be consigned to the past but are still present in everyday discrimination and structures of racism that impact on referrals to 'talking therapies'.

Thus, in our consulting rooms, the issue of 'odour' comes to be so overdetermined that we have found it difficult to find space for psychoanalytic conceptualization of this communication, above the din of already saturated social discourses.

Therapists who work with those who communicate with and via the body, especially through being 'smelly', will have come to a decision that smell is not the social taboo to which they wish to give their most emphatic response. Moral philosopher Martha Nussbaum suggests an imperative to consider how we situate ourselves in relation to these issues: 'the moral progress of society can be measured by the degree to which it separates disgust from danger and indignation, basing laws and social rules on *substantive harm*, rather than the *symbolic relationship* ... to anxieties about animality and mortality' (1999, p. 32, original emphasis). Where the broadcast of intimate odour is concerned, our response to this most personal aspect of the self is always highly political.

With thanks to Professor Forbes Morlock for consultation on this paper.

CHAPTER 5

Body odour in a psychoanalytic treatment: bridge or drawbridge to a troubled past?

Raffaella Hilty

In this chapter I explore the topic of bodily communications and somatic countertransference with a particular focus on the part played by bodily odour. In order to explore this topic, I discuss a two-year treatment with a patient who presented with a mix of borderline and narcissistic diagnostic features and a very uncomfortable symptom: an extremely strong bodily odour that I experienced as terribly unpleasant. My thesis is that the bodily odour communicated preverbal and unsymbolized experiences of early physical and emotional neglect, as well as evacuating the toxicity of those experiences. In this way it acted both as a bridge, that could help me reconstruct my patient's early traumatic past and as a drawbridge, to keep me at distance and maintain his past dissociated.

The functioning of body odour has received little attention within the psychoanalytic literature, yet this is perhaps surprising given its potential to link to the memories of early childhood experience. The connection between odour and memories has been considered by classical and contemporary authors. As Nabokov said, 'Nothing revives the past so completely as a smell that was once associated with it' (1970, p. 72) and Proust, in *Remembrance of Things Past* (1913, p. 51), is famous for capturing the way that savouring a tea-soaked madeleine put him in touch with a rich array of childhood memories. For Proust, the smell and taste of the tea-soaked madeleine acted as a symbol for those memories but, this may not be the case for patients with pre-verbal and early developmental trauma, who might have developed a rigid defence structure to remain dissociated from their troubled past. In this case even the smell of one's body, or the perceived absence of it, may act as a drawbridge to the memories of those experiences and to the possibility of their analytic reconstruction within the therapeutic relationship.

Mitrani (1995) in her discussion of Süskind's novel *Perfume: The Story of a Murderer* (1986) argues that the main character's obsession with olfactory experience illuminates a way that some patients maintain psychic survival by reliance on symptoms that speak to the earliest stages of development, which have been characterized by abuse and neglect. These symptoms point to a breakdown of psychic organization in what Ogden (1989) has described as the autistic-contiguous position, a presymbolic and sensory mode of experience, which precedes the schizo-paranoid and depressive modes described by Klein (1932), and where psychic organization is built through the experience of sensory contiguity, meaning the experience of sensory surfaces touching one another, especially the experience of the skin surface. The development of a normal autistic-contiguous psychic organization can unfold only in the relationship with the mother as a sufficiently containing object and holding environment. A breakdown of this organization leads to the implementation of autistic defences.

Individuals who experienced a failure of maternal care at this very early developmental phase could not develop what Bick (1968; 1986) called a psychic-skin, an internalization of the containing function of the object, which is introjected by sensory contact and is experienced as capable of fulfilling the function of containing the unintegrated self. The work of Anzieu (1995) on the skin-ego also illuminates how a failure of containment at this very early developmental phase may impair the development of psychical ego boundaries and the fundamental sense of one's bodily integrity. By skin-ego Anzieu refers to a mental image, based on the experience of the mother's bodily surface, that the child's ego uses to represent itself as an ego that can contain psychical contents. He explains that, 'The *infant* begins to perceive its skin as a surface when it experiences contact between its body and that of its mother, in the framework of a secure relationship of attachment to her. Through these experiences it comes to develop not only the notion of a boundary between the inside and the outside but also the confidence it will need to control its orifices, for it can only feel confident in their functions if it also has a fundamental certainty of the integrity of its bodily wrapping. In this, clinical practice confirms Bion's (1962) notion of the psychical container (…)' (1995, p. 42).

Could my patient's smell, which I experienced as extremely unpleasant, and that was uncontrollably released through the skin of his body, signify a failure at this very early stage of development? The clinical material that I am about to discuss will hopefully provide some evidence to this hypothesis.

First encounter

I will call this patient Mark. I saw Mark twice weekly in the outpatient service of a charity organization. The therapeutic treatment was undertaken face-to-face and, due to the nature of the service, our work could not be open-ended.

A colleague in the organization referred Mark to me. Mark was a 42-year-old British Caucasian man who had been adopted as an infant and had experienced psychological and physical abuse from his adoptive parents. The referral reported his main presenting symptoms as strong anxiety, depression and interpersonal difficulties. Despite these difficulties, he had managed to keep his employment steady and had been working as an accountant for many years. He was also an educated, intelligent and articulate man who had many hobbies and interests. But there was much more about Mark that caught me by surprise.

On the day of our first appointment, I went to collect him from reception. There I met a timid man who introduced himself with a weak handshake. Despite the timid way in which he introduced himself, once we arrived in the consulting room I did not need to prompt him to talk. As he began to tell me about his history and present difficulties I soon realized that I was experiencing him as somewhat polarized: both intellectually adult and emotionally chaotic. He oscillated between self-pity and contempt, sorrow and rage, at times revealing a sort of childlike demeanour which stood in sharp contrast to the physicality of a man of his age.

His narrative was fast-paced, interrupted only by short, compulsive laughs. He jumped from one topic to the other so that it was difficult for me to follow his train of thought or to consider the meaning of what he was saying. I could sense his inability to self-regulate and I noticed that he kept moving in the chair like an unsettled baby. His lack of grooming and bodily care was also apparent: his socks were mismatched, his hair looked greasy and his garments seemed dirty. I suddenly noticed that the room was beginning to fill with a very strong smell that caused me to feel disgusted, claustrophobic and unable to think. I could hardly breathe. It was as if there was not enough air for both of us in the room. At the end of the session, after he left, I realized that he had talked for almost 50 minutes and that his words, as well as his smell, had invaded the whole of the space. I felt an urge to open the window and evacuate the revolting and suffocating smell, which stayed with me for the rest of the day prompting, in my mind, a whole sequence of questions about its possible unconscious relational meaning. In my fantasy I imagined the smell coming from his feet, his greasy hair or his grubby-looking clothes. I even considered that it might come from his genitals as the odour had an acid-like quality that reminded me of cat's urine. Symbolically, I questioned whether his mother had been unable to fall in love with his bodily functions when he was an infant, leaving him for too long in his soiled nappies. Perhaps this smell was a way of communicating pre-verbal experiences of physical and emotional neglect, as well as a defence to keep me at a distance and avoid further similar experiences (Brown, 2015).

Before our second appointment I dreaded being exposed to that smell again. At the start of the session Mark began to tell me, in a highly disorganized way, the details of the chaos that he was experiencing in his flat – his flatmate had invited a friend, whom Mark hardly knew, to stay over for a few days. Once again, I noticed that the smell was filling up the room and, once more, I felt disgusted, claustrophobic and unable to think. In my mind I imagined being in a crowded, suffocating room, filled with panicking individuals who were chaotically pushing one other trying to get out. While I was listening, suspended in my own inner mental chaos, as the image that emerged in my mind clearly shows, I eventually managed to offer an intervention hoping to provide him with the containment he so desperately needed. In hindsight I think that I was also hoping to release myself from that unbearable sense of invasion that I was experiencing both mentally and somatically. I said that I could see how very difficult it was for him to manage all the chaos that the situation at home was evoking in his mind, as if his thoughts were too many and his mind too crowded. To my surprise he replied that it felt *claustrophobic*, as if there was not enough space for everybody. I added that perhaps he was feeling claustrophobic also from being in the room with me because he hardly knew me, like he hardly knew his flatmate's friend, and this might leave him feeling unsafe. The moment the claustrophobic feeling we were both experiencing was named, I regained my own mental space and I sensed that Mark had become calmer, possibly regaining his own. Even though this feeling didn't last long, I felt we had experienced a moment of connection and mutual understanding. Through an initial experience of bodily communication an image had first emerged in fantasy and it was subsequently verbalized. For the rest of the session, despite the presence of the smell, my experience of claustrophobia disappeared.

During the following days I wondered if my feeling of claustrophobia was evidence of my difficulty and subsequent refusal at receiving and tolerating some very intrusive aspects of Mark's projections. I also considered if the intensely intrusive feelings that I had experienced in my countertransference could be understood in the context of those claustrophobic phenomena that Meltzer (1992) evocatively described as a claustrum, referring to the most intrusive, rigid and controlling aspects of projective identification. This lack of psychological movement signals a stagnation of development and of coming into being as a psychologically separate individual. It is against life. One of the images that came to my mind is that of being stuck in the maternal uterus as an asphyxiating claustrum. Could the smell be an expression of the rigidity of the projective system and be seen as the link between the psychic life decay of the claustrum and the physical life decay of the body?

Relational history

During the first couple of months, Mark's relational history started to unfold. Mark was nine years old when he was told about the adoption. He recalled that on that day mother was very angry and that her rage eventually culminated in the unexpected revelation of the adoption. The words were still vivid in his mind: 'You are so bad ... of course your mother did not want you ... you are not my child, you know ...'. Father coldly confirmed the shocking revelation. The punitive and unempathic way in which the reality of the adoption was disclosed contributed to make this discovery another traumatic loss. To defend against this unbearable reality Mark used to fantasize that some day his biological mother would come back for him. I wondered in my mind, if this fantasy could be seen both as a defence against grieving the loss of a protected childhood as well as an expression of his Oedipal wish to have mother all for himself. This would help defend against the terrible blow of being excluded from the parental couple: both the biological couple who abandoned him, and the adoptive couple who could not embrace him.

Since Mark had no secure base in the family milieu to internalize, he sought for this somewhere else. His academic achievements became very important to his sense of worth and he frequently mentioned the praise of his teachers and how they encouraged him to pursue his studies. However, his wish to prove his worth through academic success was in conflict with his fear of being envied and punished. This harsh and persecutory part of himself was rooted in the experience of a punitive father who belittled his achievements and aspirations. It was this father introject, I believe, that contributed to the development of what Bion (1959, p. 314) described as an ego-destructive super-ego that attacked everything good in his life and that 'is a destroyer of the self, its relations and its objects' (O'Shaughnessy, 2015, p. 177). Mark was very attached to this critical introject and sometimes I would find myself playing this critical role in my mind. Probably this was the 'role responsiveness' (Sandler, 1976, pp. 44–5) he needed me to play so that I could become more deeply aware of his internal persecutory world.

During Mark's adolescence his father's behaviour became increasingly abusive, so much so that Mark eventually had to give up his studies. During the first stages of therapy recurrent themes were his regret for not having fulfilled his academic dreams, for not having pursued a more successful career, and a resentment and distrust for not having been believed and protected by his relatives and teachers.

First six months

Our first six months were marked by his verbal ruminations, the pervasive presence of the smell and my hatred of it. During this period I continued to reflect on the possible meaning of the smell, as it affected my ability to breathe and think properly. Bion talks about the baby's fear of dying when he experiences intolerable states of mind and explains that if the mother neglects this fear the baby becomes overwhelmed with anxiety. He calls this anxiety a 'nameless dread' (Bion, 1962, p. 309). Brown (2015) suggests that when we feel suffocated by the smell of another we are likely experiencing their own internal world of being 'choked' by their unnamed fears and anxieties. I began to speculate that through projective identification my hatred of his smell could be linked to experiencing some terrifying pre-verbal or non-symbolized experiences. This was confirmed when Mark told me that when he was a child, on several occasions, his mother threatened him with a kitchen knife. There were also other circumstances when he had experienced his parents as life-threatening. He mentioned feeling breathless when his mother punched him forcefully in the stomach or when his father held him by his throat against a wall. He recalled that when he was five years old and unwell, mother shut him outside the house on Christmas day so that he should not spoil the celebration. Mark thinks that he could have suffered severe complications had he not been guested by a compassionate neighbour. He admitted that he had never felt safe with his adoptive parents, that he often thought they wished him dead or that they had never adopted him. This made me question if he had experienced what Kahr (2007) described as an 'infanticidal attachment', where the child is exposed, either consciously or unconsciously, to death-related messages communicated by the primary caregivers. Was the fear of being killed by his parents the nameless dread that I was experiencing in my countertransference as a claustrophobic choking sensation? Could this have begun with the early abandonment by his biological parents and the nameless dread of being allowed to starve, both physically and emotionally? I can only speculate about the psychology of Mark's early infancy but it seemed that both conscious and unconscious messages of being wished dead were part of Mark's early life experience.

While interpreting the transference provided Mark with containment, I decided against directly referring to his smell, concerned that his fragile ego structure would not have allowed him to cope with the resulting feelings of shame. Moreover, I thought that any intervention about the smell at that stage might have expressed my disgust and would have imperilled our working relationship. In fact, I often questioned if any naming of the smell at that stage would have been more a retaliatory reaction from the part of me that hated this very ill part of his personality.

Winnicott (1949) in his seminal paper 'Hate in the Countertransference' explains that, even though we love and want to help our patients, we can also hate the very ill parts of them, those parts that are burdensome, needy and abusive. He compares this to how mothers love their babies but, at times, can also hate them. Babies expect absolute care from their mothers and Winnicott recognized that something so exhausting can be hate inducing. Verbalizing my hateful feelings in supervision proved to be extremely useful, as this helped me contain them while I was also processing Mark's hatred for his inner persecutory objects.

During the fifth month I had to change the time of one of our weekly sessions. This was when the intensity of the smell reached its peak. At first, Mark seemed to accept the new arrangements easily, almost compliantly. The following week, though, the smell had become stronger and I realized that this change in the therapeutic framework had left him feeling uncontained. After that session I could feel his smell on my clothes and in my whole body. It was as if I had been contaminated and infected by him. As soon as I arrived at home, I felt an urge to take a shower and put all my clothes in the washing machine. When I woke up the next day, my first thought was of his smell and I decided to go for a run hoping to sweat it out of my body. During our next session I asked Mark how he had begun to experience the new time of the therapy appointment. He was dismissive and said that he was OK with it. He told me that he was very stressed at work and that he wanted to take some days off but could not manage to do it because he felt guilty. He had also become very frustrated with a female colleague at work who used to take time off whenever she wanted. I said that he was seeing me like his colleague who takes time off whenever she wants and that I wondered if he was feeling frustrated with me because I had changed the time of our weekly session. He admitted that he would have preferred to keep the time as it was because that would have allowed him to go to some weekly social appointments. I said that I could sense he was angry with me. He replied that he knew it was not my fault. I said that he still had a right to feel angry with me. He didn't reply and I wondered if he might be afraid to lose me, had he openly expressed his anger. During the following session I realized that the smell had weakened. Perhaps the possibility of naming his anger had helped to decrease the intensity of a very primitive and concrete way of expressing it.

Throughout our first six months, Mark's narrative style continued to be very disorganized. A recurrent theme during this time was the resentment against the people who had not believed the reality of his abusive childhood experience. The reality of his experience being unacknowledged had left him with unresolved feelings of shame, rejection, distrust and a dreadful fear that his reality would disappear if his opinions were not completely mirrored by another. During these first months a lot of frustration began to emerge in connection with Mark's relational difficulties, both at work and at home. He felt consistently excluded, disbelieved and misunderstood as soon as he perceived someone else not fully agreeing with him. When someone's opinion did not neatly match his expectation Mark would be overwhelmed with fear, rather like a baby who experiences a catastrophe when he hallucinates the breast and the breast fails to appear. This was also becoming apparent in our relationship and, sometimes, the only way I could be with him was by fully mirroring his psychic reality. Britton describes the problem that these patients experience as a difficulty in 'sharing the space'. He explains that being in the same room and, symbolically, in the same psychic space, becomes a problem. Therefore, 'Instead of there being two connected independent minds, there are either two separate minds unable to connect or two people with only one mind.' (Britton 2003, p.171). My experience of Mark's body odour, as both invasive and aversive, can be seen as a primitive way of Mark expressing his difficulty in sharing psychic space, as well as the avoidance-approach dilemma typical of disorganized attachment where the source of safety is also the source of fear and anxiety.

As our first Christmas break approached, I could hear in Mark's narrative and feel in my countertransference that he was becoming increasingly angry. However, any intervention from my side that would link it to the upcoming break and touch on his narcissistic need to deny any dependence on me would be contemptuously dismissed. When we met again after the Christmas break, Mark began the session naming all the things that he was angry about, including how annoyed he was with his colleague at work who took time off whenever she liked. I said that he sounded envious of these people. I wondered aloud if he was envious of me too, as I had also taken a holiday and if, behind his frustration, he had felt not supported by me. At this point Mark almost shouted back at me saying that he had never felt supported by his parents. I said that this must have been infuriating and, also, very painful. He nodded. For the first time I felt something softening in my chest, as if the pain under his anger had come through. I think that perhaps he felt understood because, at the end of the session, for the first time, he left thanking me. It was during rare moments such as this one, when I could reach him (Stern et al., 1998), that I think he was able to make a clearer distinction in his mind between his internal persecutory objects, his present reality and me.

Second six months

After our first six months the smell had started to decrease as Mark's anger and anxiety were more frequently verbally expressed. Then, after the Easter break, he told me that he was feeling very anxious about his difficulties in managing his many social commitments. I noticed that he was subtly bringing up, once again, the change of time of one of our weekly sessions. In fact, that was the day of the week that had become an obstacle to some of his social commitments. I said that he sounded ambivalent about coming to therapy on that day of the week and that maybe he resented me for changing the time of our appointment. He finally opened up about how he truly felt. He told me that he had never wanted to change the time of our session and that I had given him no choice. He said that he had felt cheated and that, since then, he had not been able to trust me at all. My mind went blank, as if it had become flooded by the adrenaline rush of an experience of fright without solution. I eventually made an intervention. I said that, if he felt cheated by me, he must feel very unsafe to be in the room with me. As I named our shared experience of fear, I started to regain some mental space. I added that he had been let down by many people in his life and that I could understand how difficult it was for him to trust me, even though he wished he could. My intervention seemed to have contained the heightened sense of anxiety that had pervaded the room but, when Mark left, I realized that my whole body was aching. I felt no strength in my muscles. That night I dreamt of being stabbed and my dream made me think of his mother's death threats. Supervision enabled me to see that I must name these destructive attacks, which I was experiencing very vividly in my countertransference. Until then most of my interventions had helped Mark to feel contained and understood. Was it now time to help him gain insight and understanding? Patients who present a borderline and narcissistic organization may find classic intrapsychic interpretations too intrusive. Steiner (1993) contributed to bridging this problem by differentiating between what he calls 'analyst-centred interpretations' and 'patient-centred interpretations'; he explains that shifting the emphasis of the interventions on how the patient experiences the analyst can be less intrusive and help the patient feel contained and understood. However, Steiner also explains that the relief that this kind of containment brings does not necessarily lead to growth and development as it depends on the presence of the containing object. The therapist must, at times, take the risk of naming what goes on in the patient's mind, even though this may still feel challenging for the patient to tolerate. If the patient is supported in the psychic work of understanding he can eventually separate and internalize the capacity for containment and the reflective function of the therapist.

When Mark arrived at the following appointment I sensed that he was furious. He immediately told me how upset he had been since he had left the previous week. He accused me of not understanding him. He accused me again of cheating him with the change of time of our appointment. He reported my remarks from the previous week that had left him feeling misunderstood. From my point of view, they were twisted but I realized that there was no point in making another intervention. While I was struggling to keep myself regulated in my affective experience, I was also trying to mobilize my compassion so that whatever intervention I made would not come from my 'hate in the countertransference' (Winnicott, 1949) and hence be experienced as retaliatory. I reminded myself of the significance for Mark of having his reality acknowledged and I decided to let him report all of what he heard me say, so that he could feel understood. Subsequently, I shared my own experience of what I remembered saying and meant, helping him to see that what was in my mind was different from what was in his mind. I added that he seemed to feel very persecuted by me and that this was probably linked to how persecuted he had felt by his mother. My intention was to help him understand his intrapsychic reality and, at the same time, to show him that our experiences were different and could be different, that it was safe to have two separate minds and that this would not destroy our relationship. I sensed his anger building up in my body. Was this a defensive reaction because he was frightened of our minds becoming separate? I remarked that I could see how enraged he was becoming and that maybe he needed to feel enraged because this anger was making him feel potent and safe but that, underneath, he was feeling frightened. He listened silently. Then, he bent towards me and, while he was staring at me, as if he was staring into space, I felt a punch in my stomach. I was finding it almost impossible to think but, somehow, I made an intervention. I said that I could sense how angry he was and that I wondered if he wished if he could punch me. He didn't reply but eventually stopped staring at me in that almost dissociative way. Then, he sat back in the chair looking exhausted and I felt exhausted too. My countertransference had been so intense that I think, in that moment, he had experienced me concretely as his mother, rather than as if I was his mother. In hindsight I see that I had to take on that role, the role of the mother he wanted to punch and destroy, so that he could test if I would survive.

Winnicott (1969) talks about how patients who have a narcissistic or borderline personality organization have not yet made the transition between object relating and object usage. With this type of patient, the first task of therapy is to help them make this transition and to distinguish between their inner projected reality and their present external reality. He explains that if the analyst survives the attacks from the patient in the transference – attacks that are actually against the persecutory internal objects projected onto the therapist – the patient can eventually overcome his omnipotent phantasy of control over the object. In fact, he realizes that, since the object has survived his aggression, it cannot be controlled, meaning that it has not been created by him and therefore it is separate: it is real.

That session marked a shift in our relationship. When we met again Mark seemed more reflective and he reported a dream that he had the night of our last session.

Dream

> I was in Italy. I was in a house with many Italian women. I could not understand what they were saying, because I did not know the language and I was feeling uncomfortable. But I knew they were nice and caring. And then at the end of the dream I was even learning Italian.

He said that this dream must have been about me because I am Italian, and because he was in Italy with Italian women. I commented that the dream image of learning Italian could represent his wish to take in something good from me (something nice and caring) as well as his commitment to learning the language of psychoanalytic work even though, at times, this may have felt difficult and uncomfortable. After this session I wondered if the dream image of learning Italian could be seen as the unconscious confirmation of a shift in his capacity for self-reflection. Furthermore, during the following weeks Mark seemed to have become more introspective: his narrative was less chaotic, his ruminations less frequent and my experience of his smell started to be more background than foreground in our sessions.

At the end of the first year, the presence of the smell was mentioned for the first time. Mark told me that his flatmate had complained that Mark's room smelled and was very untidy. Mark said that he had never been sensitive to odour. I asked if he had experienced his parents as untidy or neglectful of his grooming when he was a child. He told me that mother used to be very tidy and obsessed with cleaning. Everything was very neat. Thinking about the possible meaning of his lack of sensitivity to odour, I questioned in my mind if his mother, who was so neat and tidy, had put into Mark all her mental toxicity and Mark was now concretely manifesting the toxicity that the relationship with his mother produced in him, while dissociating from its emotional awareness. The following session the smell seemed to have almost disappeared and he reported another dream.

Dream

I was in my room. It was clean and tidy and I was sleeping in clean white bed linen.

He explained that his room was smelly and untidy because he didn't really respect himself and that he wanted to change that. I said that since childhood he seemed to have experienced his body and mind as unworthy of respect and that this must have been very painful. I added that his lack of sensitivity to the odour that his neglectful habits were causing could be seen as a way of remaining emotionally unaware of that painful reality. We looked at the dream as an expression of his unconscious wish to change and as a confirmation of his emerging emotional awareness.

I think it is interesting that after a year of tolerating the smell this was finally named by Mark himself, as if he had reached the developmental stage for its verbal expression. The naming of the smell was linked to the experience of a mother who was 'neat and tidy' and 'very different' from him. This brought me back to the image of the mother's uterus as an asphyxiating claustrum. It left me wondering if this meaningful symptom, as well as signifying a stagnation of life development, could also be seen as an attempt to differentiate and come into being, expressing simultaneously Mark's wish and dread to be separate, a dread that was due to his fear of being engulfed or completely abandoned. These simultaneously contradictory states of mind are evidence of a lack of ego integration and differentiation and, also, of the coexistence of multiple ego states with their contradictory views of reality. Present-day attachment theory is helpful here as it describes dissociation both in the language of segregated internal working models and in disorganized attachment. It enabled me to think about the split I was perceiving between Mark's cognitive and emotional development as the result of the lack of integration of his internal working models.

Second year (first six months)

As our first summer break was approaching I noticed that the theme of exclusion had become a recurrent motif. It was present in the narrative as being left out from the life he wanted, not being believed and understood, and also being left out from the romantic units of some of his friends who were in relationships. The latter was often linked to the feelings of exclusion that he had experienced with his adoptive parents and, in my view, it must also have been strongly related to the exclusion from the biological parental couple who gave him up for adoption. In my mind I wondered if, as his smell, which was a very primitive way of communicating neglect and exclusion from the mother's mind, had decreased, his anxiety around those feelings had become now more verbalized, instead of being concretely sweated out of his body.

When we met after the summer he told me that he was happy he had this 'time off from me' and that he wished he could drop most of his commitments, including therapy, to have more time for himself. Both verbally and in my countertransference I picked up his dismissive attack and I said that he might have felt I had taken 'time off from him'. I asked if he had felt abandoned during this time and if he was now feeling angry with me and wanted to drop me to make me experience what he did. His attitude suddenly flipped. He told me, in a compliant manner, that he was only joking, that he wanted to continue therapy and that he knew perfectly well that I had not abandoned him. I saw his compliance as a defence against his fear that his anger could destroy our relationship. I told him that, even then, he still had a right to feel angry with me. After this comment he seemed calmer. He then told me about another experience when he felt he had not been understood at work and that he had been excluded by a couple of colleagues who never asked him to join them for lunch. In my mind I thought that, after giving him permission to still feel angry with me, he was reiterating that a part of him had felt excluded and abandoned by me during the summer.

During the following months his fear of being abandoned and excluded was becoming more and more verbalized but as we were getting closer to our second Christmas break, I noticed that the smell began to return both more frequently and intensely. This left me feeling confused and frustrated and, at times, hopeless that any lasting change would be possible. During these periods of apparent regression, I had to remind myself that progress is not a straight linear line but a spiralling, gradual movement. I began to think about the smell as a symptom that I hated but also as an ally. Like an image in a dream, it could help me understand whether what I was hearing on the verbal, conscious level was in line with Mark's non-verbal unconscious processes. I started to pay more attention to when the smell returned more strongly, trying to identify a pattern. I noticed that a misattunement, a progress in his ability to self-reflect, an upcoming break were all opportunities for this symptom to make its presence more noticeable. All these situations were related to separation: the real separation of a break, the emotional separation of a misattunement and the psychological separation evoked by my effort to support the development of his capacity for self-reflection.

His ambivalent feelings towards me were clearly represented by the images of two paintings that he showed me. This was in the session before the upcoming separation of our second Christmas break. He told me that he had gone to an exhibition and that he wanted to show me the pictures of his two favourite paintings. The first one was a dark geometric composition on black canvas featuring the title *Toxic Representation*. The second was a golden bas-relief featuring the title *Golden Representation*. By showing me these images, I think that Mark wanted to let me know about his struggle to hold together the love and the hate that he felt for me. In his mind he related to me with simultaneously contradictory thoughts: on one side I was the golden mother, on the other side I was the toxic mother. During the same session he recalled the day when he was shut out from the house on Christmas day. I said that he was probably feeling ambivalent towards me as he may think that I was shutting him out from my Christmas day. I pointed out that the two cards seemed to depict his ambivalent feelings but Mark dismissed any attempt from my side to explore his contradictory states of mind. My intervention, instead, seemed to have evoked his defences and, at the end of the session, I noticed that the revolting smell had, once again, filled the room.

The day we were meant to meet after Christmas he did not show up. He arrived the day after and looked puzzled when I told him that we were meant to meet the previous day. He apologized profusely and said this was not conscious. We explored some possible unconscious feelings of anger towards me for having abandoned him over Christmas. Again, he dismissed this but, half-way through the session he mentioned that a friend had killed himself. In my mind I thought that during the break he may have thought that I had died. I kept this thought for myself and I simply said that it must have been very difficult for him and that I wondered if he wished he could have been able to see me. He finally acknowledged that he had felt very angry with me because I was not there but that he also knew that this was not my fault. He thought he was constantly failing by coming to therapy feeling so angry. I said that it was very important that he could verbally express his anger while in my presence and that even if he knew it was not my fault he still had a right to feel angry.

Second year (second six months)

From a neo-Kleinian perspective, the Oedipal situation is seen as a step where the child can develop the capacity to tolerate the exclusion from the parental couple and gain a decentred perspective that leads to psychological separateness and freedom of thought (Britton, 2003). As we continued to work on his feelings of exclusion, separation and death anxiety – the ultimate separation of all – I was mindful of the importance of continuing to allow him to express his anger towards me, while also thinking and reflecting on its meaning. This was a way to support the development of his sense of agency and of working through of his resentment against his primal objects.

While a part of him was still very compliant and afraid of not meeting my expectations and the expectations of others, an emerging sense of agency started to manifest itself in some behavioural changes. I noticed that he had started to leave the consulting room opening the door and closing it behind him: previously he would rather stand waiting for me to do this for him. He was taking sick leave when he needed to. He was feeling less guilty and persecuted. He was enjoying his personal life more, having become more spontaneous and less rigid or worried. He even arrived late a couple of times, something that he had never done before and which I saw as a change in his pattern of defences. We noticed that he was feeling less fearful of being punished by me and less compelled to please me. During this period, I also made a conscious decision to decrease the frequency of my interventions, leaving him more space for self-reflection to support the development of his new emerging sense of agency. At the same time, though, things were not as 'neat and tidy' because, for example the smell had not completely disappeared. This meaningful symptom continued to return when he would experience something overwhelming, as if he needed to bring me back a smelly baby to remind me of the original maternal failure and of the part of him that still needed a lot of containment.

During the last couple of months I was mindful to name the upcoming end of therapy and explore his feelings around this. In this period he brought two dreams. In one of them he saw me crossing the street and leaving him behind, terrified of being hit by a car. In the other dream, he was frightened of being killed by a woman, a murderess whose body was covered by blood and who had blonde hair, just like me. I said that he was experiencing the upcoming end of therapy as an annihilating abandonment. I used these dreams to explore his feelings around the upcoming separation but he continued to deny any attachment to me, until our last session.

Mark arrived for our last appointment looking unexpectedly well groomed. I immediately noticed that there was no smell and that his narrative was calm and reflective. I wonder if he wanted to show me a non-smelly baby, wishing that I would not give him up for adoption. He mentioned that he had been thinking about his patterns, including his tendency to ruminate, and he explained that he had kept repeating over and over the same things because he could not trust that I would believe him. I said that I could see what he meant, as if ruminating was his way to make sure that I would hear him and believe him. He said it was a shame that he took so long to trust me. He then reported a dream that he had the previous night.

Dream

> I dreamt that I had a son and that I was giving him up for adoption. Firstly, I thought that was not good but then I felt it was OK because there was another little girl with him and they were going away together.

I asked him to repeat the dream and specifically to describe these little children. He said that his son had dark hair whereas the little girl was blonde with flowers in her hair. I asked him if he had any thoughts about the meaning of this dream and he said that he had no idea. I offered a tentative interpretation, 'I wonder if this little boy represents a part of you and refers to your own adoption? Perhaps, with the end of therapy, a part of you feels like you are being given up for adoption once again?' He stared at me in silence and I was not sure if I had said something that didn't resonate or if what I had said was a possible layer of meaning that was too painful for him to take in. So I added, 'You say that there is this blonde little girl and I can't help thinking that I am blonde'. He immediately reacted to this comment saying that this little girl had blonde hair exactly like me. I said that even if therapy had come to an end and we were facing a separation a part of him felt that he would take away a part of me. He agreed. He said that the overall feeling of the dream was a good one but that when he woke up he was feeling slightly sad. I explained that even though he was taking away something good from me he was still experiencing a separation and that it was OK to also feel sad. We acknowledged that open-ended therapy would have allowed him to continue this work and we discussed the possibility of him re-entering therapy at some point in the future. He thanked me and gave me two tickets for a photographic exhibition. He said that he got me two tickets so that I could go with someone else. I thought that he wished I would go with him but I kept this thought for myself.

Conclusions

In this chapter I have used detailed clinical material to discuss how bodily odour in the consulting room can be a powerful form of non-verbal communication which can reveal the patient's deepest emotional distress. Paying attention to my somatic countertransference, I became more and more deeply aware that the smell was an expression of embodied memories communicating traumatic experiences of early physical and emotional neglect, as well as evacuating the toxicity of those experiences. As a form of primitive bodily communication, the smell points to archaic ways of mental functioning whilst, developmentally, to a failure of the holding environment (Winnicott, 1971) at the very early stages of development. The invasive and aversive nature of the smell acted both as a bridge that could help me reconstruct my patient's traumatic past and, at the same time, as a drawbridge, that could keep me at distance and maintain his past dissociated. This can be thought of as representing the approach-avoidance dilemma typical of a disorganized attachment state of mind and of what Glasser referred to as the 'core complex' (1979, p. 278), acting both as a bridge and as a drawbridge to attachment and relating.

Looking back, my clinical work with Mark has been one of the most dreaded and, at the same time, most rewarding experiences I have had. Although many years have passed, his memory is still vivid in my mind. Working with him sparked what, at that time, was a newly born interest in bodily communications in psychotherapy and, for this, I am particularly grateful. Regretfully our work could not be open-ended. Nevertheless, after only two years I had noticed in Mark some significant changes, such as a decrease of the frequency and intensity of the smell as well as of the intensity of the transference and countertransference. I also noticed an improved ability to relate to me, for example by acknowledging my absence and missing my support at times of separation, as well as being able to experience sadness in my presence when we had to say goodbye.

All of this can be seen both as a shift in the use of primitive defences and of an increased ability to differentiate more adequately, at an unconscious level, between phantasy and reality.

NOTE TO THE READER

This chapter is based on a prior publication of the author in the British Journal of Psychotherapy.

All names have been changed and any verbatim or specific content that would make the patient recognizable has been altered to maintain confidentiality.

CHAPTER 6

In corpore inventitur: embodied countertransference and the process of unconscious somatic communication

Salvatore Martini

Due to the unconscious pressures deriving from strong defence mechanisms manifested by some of my patients I have frequently come into contact with the experience that Jung (1921, pp. 294–5) referred to as *participation mystique* and have therefore had the possibility to observe the varying ways it manifests during the therapeutic process. These can take the form of unpleasant and embarrassing bodily sensations, such as severe muscle tension and physiological urges.

Together with Jung's closely related concepts of 'unconscious identity' and 'psychic infection', Rosemary Gordon (1965, p. 128) equated *participation mystique* with the primitive defence mechanism of projective identification. This can pass on vital information regarding the early onset and degree of severity of the patient's psychological damage, above all when somatic reactions arise in the analyst.

The particular localizations of these countertransferential phenomena in the analyst's body often seem to be symbolically connected to the patient's specific psychological problems. This primal communicative dimension, where the body becomes the 'intermediary of the encounter' (Callieri, 2007, p. 153), opens up the opportunity for a profound interaction between the patient and the therapist, leading to a possible activation of archetypal energies, which are active in the depths of the psyche. I am therefore convinced that it is necessary for the therapist to understand

and explore the phenomenon of embodied countertransference and the way it can be used as a means of analytic investigation. Such an approach is receptive to multifaceted psychic contents and facilitates multiple levels of communication, which can expand and enrich the dialogue between patient and therapist.

Embodied countertransference as an 'organ of information'

In his book *The Psychoanalytic Process* Donald Meltzer states that 'conviction about analytical theory can only come from experience; each analyst, guided by teachers and the literature, must "discover" the whole of analysis by himself.' (Meltzer, 1967, p. xvi). During my training as an analyst at the Italian Association of Analytical Psychology (AIPA), I was always aware that in order to truly practice this profession I would inevitably find myself having to deal with the psychological suffering solicited by the painful thoughts and experiences of my patients. Nevertheless, I never imagined that these feelings would manifest so frequently in corporeal ways, even in the form of acute physical pain. As Kradin points out, 'analytical training generally provides little guidance' for achieving 'somatic empathy' (Kradin, 2011, p. 43). Samuels also affirms that even an 'accurate analytical training' cannot fully prepare one for the experience of countertransference (Samuels, 2013, p. 1).

I might have understood more clearly what was in store for me if I had connected the separate affirmations made, over the years, by leading psychoanalysts on the theme of countertransference. After many years of professional experience, I eventually came to see them as intimately related to each other, also thanks to the fact that many of these authors consistently use the word 'organ' when referring to unconscious communications between the patient and the analyst.

This shared term can be traced back to 1929 with Jung, who defined the propensity to be influenced by the patient as an 'organ of information', which has a fundamental role within the therapeutic relationship (Jung, 1929, para. 163). Three decades later, while describing 'syntonic countertransference', Michael Fordham (1960, p. 247) defined the analyst's unconscious as an 'organ of information' or a 'perceptual system', although – in an exchange of papers with Schwartz-Salant in the

Journal of Analytical Psychology (Fordham, 1991; Schwartz-Salant, 1991) – he warned against an incautious use of embodied countertransference in analysis. Then, in 1962, Bion described the mother's faculty of *rêverie* as the 'receptor organ for the infant's harvest of self-sensation' (Bion, 1962, p. 308). In 1969 Meltzer defined countertransference as an 'organ of consciousness' (Meltzer, 1967, p. xii) and finally, in a ground-breaking paper on embodied countertransference, Andrew Samuels – taking his cue from Corbin (1972) – defined it as 'an organ of visionary knowledge' (Samuels, 1985, p. 61).

The fact that these authors, each with their own distinct theoretical approaches, use the word 'organ' to refer to the analyst's countertransference could be seen as a mere coincidence. Instead I believe that they all intuitively felt that it was the most effective way to express what happens when the analytical dyad comes into being, making it practically impossible to effect a clear separation between psyche and soma. As Jung affirms, 'Psyche is as much a living body as body is living psyche: it is just the same.' (Jung, 1989, p. 114). He describes a *psychoid* realm, a 'unitary world' (Jung, 1958, para. 852) that cannot be directly represented, 'where instinct predominates' (Jung, 1947–54, para. 380), and where the psychic and somatic spheres co-exist. Here we can encounter 'a psyche that touches matter ... and, conversely, a matter with a latent psyche' (Jung, 1947–54, para. 441). During his second seminar at the Tavistock Clinic on 1 October 1935, while answering a question by Bion, Jung explained that, 'The two things, the psychic fact and the physiological fact, come together in a particular way ... we see them as two on account of the utter incapacity of our mind to think of them together.' (Jung, 1935, para. 135) Jung saw this correspondence of mind and body as inherent to 'the real nature of the archetype' (Jung, 1947–54, para. 417), and Fordham similarly defined it as 'a psychosomatic entity having two aspects' one of which is 'linked closely with physical organs, the other with unconscious and potential psychic structures' (Fordham, 1969, p. 96).

I intend to explain how, within what I have defined elsewhere as 'the process of embodied communication' (Martini, 2016, p. 10), the analytic dyad can enter this psychoid area thanks to the initial somatic reactions of the therapist. These constitute a manifestation of the split-off complexes of the patient, and can guide the analytic couple to share in a progressive transition from a complexual to an archetypal level.

I believe that the therapist's individual sensations of embodied countertransference mirror the inability of the patient's consciousness to accommodate unelaborated affective elements. They are the result of the patient's defensive attempts to reject and repel psychic contents that are so frightening that they threaten to overwhelm his/her conscious mind and that his/her 'thought thinking apparatus' is utterly incapable of elaborating (Bion, 1962, p. 306).

The analyst's somatic sensations during the analytic session are closely linked to the patient's primitive defence mechanisms of mind/body splitting and projective identification. Mind/body splitting arises as a protection from non-mentalizable somatic sensations within a primary relationship that is deficient and dominated by particularly aggressive and frustrating separation anxieties. The child's consequent inability to establish a connection between affects and bodily sensations can eventually lead him to erect a structure of rigid psychic functioning with a defensive role. This is often accompanied by an unyielding barrier which protects him from the suffering of painful affects, but also prevents him from recognizing the corresponding emotions, and even from desiring or imagining anything that might be genuinely pleasant or fulfilling. The incapacity to represent one's inner states leads to an all-pervasive sense of existential emptiness, helplessness and impotence, which seems unresolvable and insurmountable (Caretti, 2006).

Patients affected by a mind/body splitting tend to stimulate somatic reactions in the analyst and to suffer from a dearth of vigour defined by Wiener as 'disturbances in vitality' (Wiener, 1994, p. 345) and by Connolly as the 'sense of deadness' (Connolly, 2013, p. 642). This is the fatal consequence of the fact that 'the mother at a very early stage, and often the father at later stages, may have failed to engage with and to mirror back' to the child 'the aliveness of his or her body' (Connolly, 2013, p. 644). As Clark points out, 'When the environment (mother/parent) fails ... the unmediated physical and emotional distress becomes so great that the psyche dissociates from the persecuted soma' (Clark, 1996, p. 356).

Newton and Clark refer to mind/body splitting as a failure to constitute what Winnicott called a 'psycho-somatic partnership' (Newton, 1965, p. 152; Clark, 1996, p. 356). Mara Sidoli also underlines how this condition can result from an early emotionally disturbed or traumatic relationship with mothers who were 'unable to mediate violent archetypal affective discharges in their infants' (Sidoli, 2000, p. 104). McDougall affirms that mind/body splitting occurs in early infancy when 'separation and difference are feared as experiences that may destroy the sense of self' (McDougall, 1989, p. 42), while Modell points out that the mother's 'insensitivity to the contours and outlines of the child's sense of self and autonomy' – a by-product of her denial that there is any difference between them – can lead to a permanent mind/body split in the child (Modell, 1990, p. 105). He also affirms that this condition results in a persistent 'schizoid defence of non-communication' and a frequent recourse to projective identification (Modell, 1990, p. 106).

The archaic defence mechanism of projective identification was elucidated for the first time by Melanie Klein in her 1946 essay 'Notes on Some Schizoid Mechanisms'. She defines projective identification as an unconscious fantasy by which the newborn child eliminates the psychic suffering induced by unfamiliar and as yet unknown somatic sensations and bodily pains by splitting and projecting them onto the mother, with the unconscious aim of possessing and controlling her. It is worth bearing in mind that Klein 'was punctilious about specifying the exact physical means by which a projection was being effected and into which part of the recipient's body.' (Bott Spillius,1988, p. 84).

This concept was then gradually elaborated and extended by several post-Kleinian psychoanalysts (Bion, 1959; Rosenfeld, 1971; Grotstein, 1981; Joseph, 1987; Meltzer, 1992). Bion was the first to attribute a communicative function to the mechanism of projective identification, thereby going beyond Klein's conception that it merely served to evacuate states of anguish – bodily in the initial stages of infantile development and then mental – and in this way he made a vital contribution to our understanding of mother-child dynamics. Bion pointed out that the mother accepts, contains and digests these contents by means of her faculty of *rêverie* and then gives them back to the child in a mitigated and more tolerable form. His 'container-contained' model and his novel concept of *rêverie* offered a theoretical-clinical explanation of unconscious child–mother communication, which he also equated with analogous aspects of the patient–analyst relationship.

Projective identification thus not only involves attempts to eject or expel painful affective contents but may also, as Modell affirms, constitute 'a persistent and chronic form of communication between analyst and analysand' which is 'analogous to the automatic physiological defenses of the body' (Modell, 1990, p. 56). This mechanism is not just a defence system for avoiding psychic pain, but it also constitutes an unconscious attempt to induce the suffering of the patient in the analyst (Stone, 2006, p. 111). Thus the analyst has the task of working on his or her own embodied countertransference, in order to transform the drastic splitting activated by the patient into a healthy body–psyche integration, and then to help him/her to gradually acknowledge and elaborate his/her psychic pain.

The authors of the book *Shared Realities – Participation Mystique and Beyond* (2014) put the Jungian concept of *participation mystique* in relation to the mechanism of projective identification. In his chapter Marcus West points out that '*participation mystique* takes a much broader brushstroke approach' than projective identification, and that in the context of unconscious communication between patient and analyst it 'lays bare the underlying dynamics more clearly' (West, 2014, p. 57). The several authors of the book provide diverse descriptions of this unconscious phenomenon, which hint at its elusive, shifting and kaleidoscopic nature and indicate that it can arise in many different ways, moments and situations during analysis.

I would claim that *participation mystique* is constantly present also during the process of unconscious somatic communication, during which it manifests with similar unpredictable variations in its form and intensity. This ongoing process of interaction between patient and analyst can be divided into three different phases, each with its own particular modalities of manifestation. They occur during analysis not only in a linear and progressive manner, but also in non-linear and oscillatory ways, mingling with each other, and rising or diminishing in intensity depending on the therapeutic dyad's capacity to tolerate closeness, intimacy and psychic pain at each specific moment during analysis. These three different aspects of embodied countertransference can be defined as follows: an impediment to the imaginative capacity of the analyst; a communication of split-off complexes of the patient; and finally a mechanism on the archetypal level, which becomes the 'creative source of an interaction beyond the powers of the conscious personality' (Schwartz-Salant, 1982, p. 108).

In an attempt to clearly illustrate these three phases I intend to refer to the specific case of a patient of mine, who I will refer to as 'Emanuele'. He was in his early twenties at the start of analysis and was suffering from severe anxiety attacks and serious intestinal disturbances. Both his parents were deaf-mute, although he himself had no kind of hearing impairment.

The beginning of the alchemical opus: the *Nigredo*

In the initial phase of analysis, projective identification pulls the analyst down into the dark and undifferentiated unconscious realm that Jung associated with the alchemical process of the *Nigredo*. He writes that the therapist 'has as much difficulty in distinguishing between the patient and what has taken possession of him as has the patient himself' (Jung, 1946, para. 375). The mechanism of projective identification is used by the patient in a defensive manner in order to discharge or unload his/her unthinkable and threatening affects. The patient unconsciously feels that the contents of his/her split-off complexes are a threat to the conscious mind, which is incapable of elaborating or digesting them, and they are therefore expelled into the analyst's body. In this way the analyst's faculty of symbolic thinking is blocked, preventing any kind of fruitful or helpful contact between patient and therapist. The analyst experiences 'a somatic symptom of a dissociated affect, inaccessible to the employment of schizoid mechanisms' and his/her 'elaboration is blocked, somewhat like a frozen computer, and the development of thought is impossible' (Carvalho, 2014, p. 374). Hilty states that the intensity of the somatic projective identification renders the analyst 'unable to think' (Hilty, 2020, p. 203), and West points out that this incapacity of the patient's mind 'relates primarily to the fact that affect associated with the original trauma is so powerful that it disrupts thinking' (West, 2014, p. 59).

Nevertheless these embodied affects can very effectively reveal the defensive dissociative mechanisms of the patient and that he or she 'is temporarily leaving the here and now' (Schwartz-Salant, 1982, p. 125). The disorientating capacity of unconscious communication to drag the analyst into the interior dimension of the analysand can therefore have positive implications, if the therapist manages to endure and contain these burdensome and oppressive manifestations of the patient's split-off contents. The analyst needs to take them upon himself/herself and bear their weight, with the faith that his/her understanding will eventually 'germinate' (Samuels, 1985, p. 54), and trusting that the patient will one day be able to consciously elaborate these contents. Lemma, taking her cue from Lombardi and Pola (2010) and Ferro (2003), refers to this as 'the analyst's sensory acceptance of the patient's projection', which is 'an essential prerequisite before interpretation can be helpful' (Lemma, 2015, p. 115).

Emanuele is a tall youth with a burly body, and he surprises me right away with a radiant smile in striking contrast with his bewildered and sad gaze. When he introduces himself and takes my hand in a soft grip, I get the impression that his big body is actually rather weak and lacking in vitality. During our first session Emanuele tells me that he had asked for psychological help after spending a sleepless night, terrified by 'the background noise of silence', which made him feel he was going mad. He describes it as a 'deafening and continuous sound' that ever since then has disturbed his sleep and his peace of mind. When he tells me that his parents are both deaf it occurs to me that this fact must be connected in some way to the disturbing and frightening sound of silence, which he talks about incessantly for the whole duration of our exploratory consultation session. I repeatedly try to change the subject and ask him about his life, in the hope of creating a case history, but all these attempts are in vain. In fact he doesn't even seem to hear my questions.

While Emanuele drones on, endlessly repeating himself, I start to feel more and more detached and alienated. The session seems to be lasting far longer than the usual hour and his voice starts to sound like distant and muffled background noise. I eventually give up trying to redirect the conversation and start to feel impatient and uncomfortable, without consciously connecting these feelings to the session. Finally, when the interminable hour is over, Emanuele thanks me in an excessively obsequious and formal way and leaves, but my free-floating malaise remains, becoming more intense and concrete, taking the form of an intense feeling of nausea. It is only then that I realize that my attempts to change the subject of the discourse were connected with my unpleasant sensations. I start to appreciate how complex our encounter has been and I attempt to reconstruct and understand my countertransferential experience.

During the following sessions Emanuele talks about more general aspects of his life, but I am assailed ever more intensely and frequently by sensations of nausea, every time he indulges in meticulous and obsessive descriptions of the smallest details of his daily routines. At the end of these four exploratory sessions we agreed to meet twice a week. Emanuele's analysis would last for a total of six years. It was only after nine months of analysis that I managed to break through the barrier of apparently empty and meaningless noise that he had obstinately erected and, for the first time since the start of our sessions, I cautiously made an initial interpretation of his possible feelings in relation to analysis, which soon led to the therapeutically valuable results that I will describe below.

Emanuele's incessant monologues were an unconscious attempt to construct a wall of words that saturated our sessions and put himself at a safe and reassuring distance from the therapeutic experience, so that he could control and block it. Susanna Wright's words are particularly relevant here: 'Perhaps from a wish to stay in control of his experience, perhaps as one way of keeping my analytical intervention safely at bay, the day to day accounts of his life did not encourage much empathic engagement' (Wright, 2020, p. 540).

Ogden defines this apparent attempt to sabotage the analytic relationship as a necessary defence against the primordial anxiety of 'dissolution of boundedness' (Ogden, 1989, p. 81), which tends to create what Bick (1968) called a 'second skin formation' of a psychological and interpersonal type. This defence is prevalent in patients suffering from early relational trauma, who have the typical schizoid defences arising from a failure to overcome the 'autistic-contiguous mode'. Ogden considers this as the primary pre-symbolic and sensory-dominated form of psychological organization, which is operative from the very first moment of life (Ogden, 1989, p. 48–50).

With the benefit of hindsight, I now believe that the nausea I felt so intensely in the initial sessions must have been a strong countertransferential reaction on my part, resulting from the patient's projective identifications which also had a significant communicative component, in apparent contrast to the defensive mechanisms he was constructing at the same time. My physical reactions of retching, the expression of a need for ejection, thus indicate that I had come into contact with a strongly split-off complex similar to 'a sort of body' with its own physiology which 'can upset the stomach' (Jung, 1935, para. 149). Jung affirms that the act of eating is symbolically connected to the assimilation of complexes (Jung, 1930, p. 19). In this sense my countertransferential bodily experiences may have reflected Emanuele's inability to integrate affective contents which were unconsciously threatening and disturbing. I started to realize that I was dealing with a patient who, despite his apparent willingness and openness to enter into the analytic process, also had a strong unconscious resistance to taking this step. However, by means of unconscious communications through projective identification, he was also summoning me to make a commitment to the unconscious therapeutic relationship that was deep, but also dark, disturbing and destabilizing. In this regard Jung writes that the 'paradoxical blend of positive and negative, of trust and fear, of hope and doubt, of attraction and repulsion, is characteristic of the initial relationship' (Jung, 1946, para. 375).

When the analyst eventually becomes aware of the fact that he has been drawn into the psychic dynamics of the *Nigredo* he is at last able to put the right distance between himself and the patient's projections. It is only then that it is possible to start out on the genuine therapeutic journey that the patient unconsciously perceives as the route to recovery. The analyst needs to develop a sort of all-embracing understanding that starts from his/her somatic symptoms, inductively giving them a broader meaning and a deeper value, that can help him/her to get in touch with the deep anguish of the analysand. Projective identifications need to be transformed into a means for encouraging the analytic process, thanks to which the patient can start to elaborate his inner suffering and recognize his defensive mechanisms.

It is worth bearing in mind that, upon experiencing forms of embodied countertransference, the analyst must be able to respect and protect the patient's corresponding dissociative reactions, as in certain moments during the therapeutic process they have the important function of preserving the integrity of the patient's ego-complex. They can also ensure the survival of the analytic relationship itself, by safeguarding the patient's consciousness from the anguish arising from unthinkable thoughts (Connolly, 2013, p. 651). The failure to safeguard these defences can in effect retraumatize the patient, with the analyst acting in the role of an intrusive parent who is not in tune with the child's needs and feelings. To avoid this danger the patient can react by abandoning therapy, for reasons that he is unable to consciously understand or elaborate. This might in fact be the lesser evil since the analyst's ongoing incapacity to understand how to deal with the situation can reinforce the patient's defences, instead of helping him to enter into a shared therapeutic process. In some cases the patient can even suffer from severe somatic reactions due to premature interventions that he is not yet prepared to face.

As I have mentioned, nine months after the start of analysis there was an important development which, thanks to a partial relaxation of the patient's defences, allowed me to finally glimpse the possibility of establishing a deeper connection. When he enters the consulting room

Emanuele tells me that today he hasn't thought of anything to talk about, as he usually does before our sessions. He says that he needs to feel relaxed and, seeing that his body appears to be even more rigid than normal, I invite him to lie down on the couch. After he does so Emanuele starts to talk with an energetic voice that instantly grabs my attention, as it is so different from the monotonous tone with which he normally delivers his stultifying over-detailed monologues. He tells me that his father frequently gets up at night to make sure that the gas-tap in the kitchen is turned off.

> **Emanuele:** Nobody has ever talked about it at home, but it's something he's always done. I don't understand why we can't talk about it. Nobody talks about it. Why is that? (long pause) It's as if he's unable to stay lying down. He has to get up to check and control the situation.

> **Me:** Maybe it's also difficult for you to stay lying down and talk about these things now. You might feel you can't control the situation. Perhaps deciding what you want to talk about before coming here is your way of controlling emotions in our relationship?

Emanuele immediately dismisses this as a psychologist's 'absurd habit of searching for meaning even in quite irrelevant phrases', but he then proceeds to talk about his own obsessive tendency to meticulously check that the water taps at home are turned off due to his fear that their seals and gaskets might break. I realize that the transition to the couch, and my suggestion that he might be trying to control his destabilizing feelings, have sparked off, first of all, a description of his father's obsessive rituals, and then an account of his own fears, making it possible for us to engage in more spontaneous interactions and intense exchanges.

In fact, during our next session, he tells me he has dreamt of an angry dog unleashed inside an underground enclosure. A thick glass wall separated him from this rabid dog, which started barking and growling at him as soon as it noticed him. Emanuele says that, 'It almost seemed that he wanted to devour me.' While he speaks I see this dream as an effective representation of Emanuele's feelings of anger and envy in reaction to my attempt, during the previous session, to approach his internal world with my tentative interpretation of his emotions and of his defensive attitude towards our analytic encounters. His mention of his fear that the water gaskets might break had already indicated that he had started to perceive the weakening of his psychic defences, which filled him with dread.

In the words of Eulert-Fuchs, 'Individuals in whom representations aren't formed often appear to be standing behind a glass wall. Because the limited symbolic processing leads to a lack of a vivid contact with their inner as well as the external world, they have to build a barrier against overwhelming impressions from within and from outside' (Eulert-Fuchs, 2020, p. 155). A few days after the session it became clear to me that the glass wall probably also represented the separation between Emanuele's visual and acoustic perceptions, due to his long-standing difficulties in communicating with his deaf parents. This situation may have contributed to the formation of a mind/body splitting and to a 'lack of coordination' between stimuli and affects (Clark, 1996, p. 356), leading to an inability to coherently elaborate and comprehend the events of his life and the emotions associated with them. As we shall see, the theme of the dog would reappear in a dream Emanuele had more than two years later, in another form that was not so immediately obvious or easy to recognize.

The second phase: body babblings and the borderline of Hermes

The manifestations of embodied countertransference in the analyst are sometimes the harbingers of profound psychic experiences that the analytic couple will experience during the course of analysis. If the analyst is able to receive and accept the patient's projections and grasp the communicative value of his/her own somatic reactions, the second phase of the process of somatic communication can begin, through the medium of the *subtle body*. Jung (1946, para. 454) defines it as 'an *anima media natura*', a 'middle thing [...] which is spirit as well as body' (Jung 1989, p. 432), and according to Stone (2006, p. 112) it is 'an intermediate space between the analyst and patient'. Jung suggests that it can act as a sort of conduit for unconscious somatic and psychic communications within the therapeutic dyad. He describes the subtle body as 'the definite abode of what old philosophy would have called an *entelechia*, the thing which tries to realize itself in existence' (Jung, 1930, p. 116). It is here that interpersonal messages are able to attain the natural potential inherent in human relationships, which are indispensable for the progress of the ego in relation to the Self. 'Relationship to the self is at once relationship to our fellow men', as Jung affirms (Jung, 1946, p. 234).

In his seminars on Nietszche's Zarathustra, Jung makes a clear distinction between the psychic unconscious and the somatic unconscious, affirming that the Self has a somatic as well as a psychic aspect, and that the physical body constitutes its external manifestation (Jung, 1989, p. 403). He also refers to an impulse of the Self that is incarnated in the body, saying that if this impulse is obstructed for any reason, the Self tends to manifest in a dysfunctional manner with negative somatic symptoms (Jung, 1989, p. 404). Thus the 'body babblings' of the analyst described by Schwartz-Salant (1982, p. 125) can be understood as a countertransferential manifestation of the embodied impulse of the patient's Self. These particular somatic symptoms arise from the patient's inability to perceive, due to his splitting, the individuative urges that arise from his body.

With the help of the physical sensations within his own body, which mirror the patient's dissociative defences, the analyst can effect a mind-body unification through her/his embodied *rêverie*. Within this dream-like state that Wright (2020, p. 553) calls the 'dreaming mind', and that De Rienzo (2021, p. 262) defines as a 'semi-hallucinatory elaboration', the analyst can connect and combine the spontaneous mental images that s/he experiences, as well as any bodily symptoms, with the psychic contents that have been split from the patient's consciousness.

In order for the embodied *rêverie* to occur it is necessary for the analyst to believe and trust in the possibility of unconscious communication, and to have the courage to abandon the safe limits of consciously understanding everything that happens in analysis. Marc Winborn (2014, p. 81) in the context of an investigation into the theme of *participation mystique*, points out that 'entering into *rêverie* is not a light switch, to be turned on and off at will'. It is essential to reach what López-Pedraza calls 'the borderline of Hermes' (López-Pedraza, 1977, p. 13) and to linger there, letting one's somatic perceptions function as 'omens' that can facilitate 'a hermetic connection between the psychological events and the body' (López-Pedraza, 1977, p. 40). Hermes was the god of wayfarers and marker-stones (López-Pedraza, 1977, p. 3), and the physical symptoms of the analyst can similarly be seen as significant milestones on the analytic journey, as well as the harbingers of potential 'moments of meeting' (Stern et al., 1998, p. 913) between patient and analyst. Wiener (2004, p. 164) defines such moments as 'intersubjective unconscious experiences' that can facilitate change as much as, or even more than, the therapist's verbal interpretations. Thus the analyst's capacity to perceive with both the body and mind can help the therapeutic couple to recognize and activate the 'interactive nature of the analytic relationship, in which the Self of the patient and that of the analyst influence each other consciously and unconsciously' (Wiener, 2004, p. 171).

During a session shortly before the Christmas vacation, two years after the beginning of analysis, Emanuele tells me of his latest dream, in which he was eating a hot dog. He then starts to describe his passion for this food in his usual detailed manner, telling me that he once ate so many hot dogs that he felt ill and vomited. Suddenly I am assailed by an intense sensation of nausea that reminds me of what I felt during the first exploratory sessions. Fortunately it subsides after a while, being progressively replaced by a drowsy torpor. Emanuele's voice starts to sound distant and muted, and I remember a hot summer afternoon when my wife and I enjoyed some hot dogs in Central Park, New York, during our honeymoon.

This mental pleasant image is then abruptly replaced by that of a dog's erect penis. The shock instantly wakes me from my stupor and I mentally translate 'hot dog' literally into the Italian term 'cane caldo'. The dream of the barking dog that Emanuele had recounted over a year before comes to mind. My attention returns to Emanuele and I am surprised to hear that he is telling me about a holiday he had in New York. I ask him if he remembers his dream about the angry dog, and jokingly point out that this time he dreamt of a 'cane caldo'. He is clearly amused by this connection.

Emanuele: It's true, I wonder why they call it that – a 'hot dog'. In the other dream it was an angry dog.

Me: It was angry because you'd got too close to it.

Emanuele: It was absolutely furious.

Me: Do you ever get angry when someone gets too close to you?

After a pause Emanuele starts to speak more slowly and reflectively.

Emanuele: My father gets too close to me. He comes into my room without knocking. He intrudes into my personal spaces ... My mother is cold and unfeeling, my father hugs me and kisses me. ... I remember I was very small ... I was lying on the bed and I was naked. ... Dad showed me how to touch myself. He spoke to me with sign language and made an up and down hand gesture. ... Maybe he just wanted to show me how I should wash myself, but at that time I thought he was showing me how to masturbate, so I began to think he was gay.

In this analytical exchange we can consider my sleepy torpor as an important embodied countertransferential phenomenon; a state described in detail by several psychoanalysts (Field, 1989; Ogden, 1994; Devescovi, 2009; Connolly, 2013; Lemma, 2015; Wright, 2020). I now believe that my drowsiness may not have arisen from Emanuele's defences, so much as from our unconscious attempt to establish the right distance between each other. Once we had finally managed to find this well-balanced and safe shared space we were able to enter a state of *rêverie* that opened up a new phase in our analysis. This state of somnolent intimacy, like that of the mother and child, can lead to a deep and significant contact between the analyst and patient. In fact it brought me in touch with Emanuele's traumatic childhood experiences of an emotionally distant mother and a disturbingly intrusive father. The fact that verbal communication was impossible with his mother and father, and that she was so lacking in empathy and feeling, accounts for Emanuele's difficulty in associating his emotions appropriately and coherently with his sensory perceptions.

The dream of the angry dog, triggered off by my attempt to interpret his feelings, reveals his repressed anger and concealed resentment towards his intrusive father. Rather than realistically elaborating his true interactions with his parents, Emanuele had evidently distorted his life experiences through the lens of unconscious fantasies. The dream of the hot dog was no doubt activated by our increasingly close relationship, and seems to be an expression of unconscious erotic fantasies that boys usually direct towards their mother, but that Emanuele had projected onto his father, the only parent who actually tried to communicate with him.

My recurrent nausea may have been due to the inability of the patient's psychic system to contain and elaborate his traumatic childhood experiences and the somatic disturbances that they had generated. Moreover, my initial countertransferential nausea foreshadowed Emanuele's difficulties in consciously 'digesting' the distressing intrusion into consciousness of homosexual fantasies regarding the figure of the father-therapist (as would in fact happen a year later, as I will recount in due course).

The third phase: the *Coniunctio*

The analytic dyad has the difficult task of properly interpreting and directing unleashed inarticulate energies arising from the reconnection with 'split-off, schizoid sectors of the psyche, sectors in which Oedipal and pre-Oedipal sexuality – the latter containing archetypal or impersonal sexual energies – are contained along with intense frustrations and despair.' (Schwartz-Salant and Stein, 1984, p. 8). It is therefore necessary for both the patient and the analyst to deal with problematic and confusing somatic sensations that can be all too easily rejected, misunderstood, or even equated with arousal of a sexual nature (Field, 1989; Connolly, 2013). In these cases the analyst must be able to effectively channel the powerful energies activated by therapy, thereby replacing the inadequate or dysfunctional modalities that the patient's parents had enacted towards their child. The analyst thus has to conceive of sexuality 'in terms of impersonal archetypal connections' (López-Pedraza, 1977, p. 13).

The 'reconciliation of opposites' (Jung, 1989, p. 433) – consisting of psyche and matter, the two poles of the archetype of the Self – initially effected by the analyst, by means of his embodied *rêverie*, can give rise to the *Coniunctio*, the third phase of the process of somatic communication. Patient and analyst experience the union of two separate individuals and are thus put in touch with the life-giving energies of the collective unconscious. In this realm, defined by Schwartz-Salant (1989, p. 131) as the 'third area', we encounter what Jung described as 'kinship libido … the core of the whole transference phenomenon' (Jung, 1946, para. 445). This fundamental drive guides the individual towards deep human relationships, as a necessary condition for gaining access to the primal structuring dimension of the collective unconscious. Once this has been achieved, the frozen process of individuation, finally freed from hindrances, can be reactivated and sustained.

As Schwartz-Salant points out, within this third field 'two people can apprehend a variety of linking structures, notably fusion, distance and union' (Schwartz-Salant, 1989, p. 110). The dynamics of the primordial stage of the mother–child relationship recur in this area of a psychoid type, charged with unsuspected therapeutic possibilities. The analytic dyad enters into contact with this 'basic matrix' by becoming a 'two-person unit' (Carvalho, 2014, p. 9; Newton, 1965, p. 153) where 'everything is everything else' (Carvalho, 2014, p. 371). In this interactive field, according to Neumann, patient and analyst can have 'an emotionally toned unitary experience' entailing a 'reciprocal co-ordination between world and psyche' thanks to the 'archetypal structures which embrace both' (Neumann, 1949, p. 27). Thus the analytic couple can gain access to the psyche's self-healing capacity, which consists in 'organizing and shaping elements of an instinctual or imaginal character' (Addison, 2019, p. 35), as a necessary condition for reactivating the patient's process of individuation.

Emanuele's separation anguish and the consequent somatic reactions in his body and my own were often intensified when there was an interruption in our sessions. Almost exactly a year after the hot dog dream, in the last session before the Christmas holidays, Emanuele tells me that the previous week he had at last plucked up the courage to invite a girl to see the film *Vincere* – literally 'to win' – at the cinema. He seems happy and gratified at this new development, and I too feel a certain sense of approval, almost like paternal pride, mingled with satisfaction that his analysis is finally yielding some concrete and positive results. However, he then sheepishly adds that he was so terrified of soiling himself that he inserted a cork into his anus. My feelings of satisfaction are immediately replaced by dismay, leaving me demoralized and disheartened.

Emanuele: I didn't enjoy the film at all. (Long pause) I don't know why but, even though I'd tried so hard, I'm not so happy about how the evening went.

Me: Perhaps 'vincere' in those conditions was not such a victory for you.

He seems deeply affected by what I have said and he sighs deeply. We both immerse ourselves in our thoughts. The session ends with us both united by a long intensely pregnant silence.

In the first session after the Christmas holidays, Emanuele confesses to me that he has had a strange and embarrassing thought. After some hesitation he tells me that after our previous session he was very 'affected by what we said'. He then went home in a state of arousal and watched an online porn video in which a female psychologist had sex with a patient. He hesitantly adds, 'I had the fantasy that I was possessing you, Doctor.'

I am left speechless by this utterly unexpected confession, and Emanuele starts talking to fill the embarrassing silence. It occurs to me that it is thanks to the good level of trust, which we have established, that he has been able to tell me about this homoerotic fantasy. I recall the Jungian concept of 'symbolic homosexuality' (Jung, 1930, p. 489), which allows me to go beyond the simplistic idea that he might have homoerotic tendencies. Instead it seems that the kinship libido connected with the intense intimacy that we had experienced in the previous session had stimulated a state of sexual arousal that was difficult for him to elaborate. The analytic couple was evidently starting to deal with the unconscious sexual fantasies that had distorted Emanuele's interpretation of his overly intrusive father's attitudes towards him, and distorted his perception of the son/father (and patient/analyst) interaction.

When my attention returns to what Emanuele is saying, I realize that he is once more describing his intestinal disturbances when he attempts to socialize with attractive girls. He tells me that diarrhoea is no longer a problem, although he still has painful stomach cramps. At that moment I feel a rapidly increasing abdominal pain immediately followed by an intense need to defecate. I desperately try to restrain this impulse by contracting my anal sphincter, which leads to an intense pang of pain. I am about to excuse myself and head for the bathroom, when I realize that I must stay seated and try to contain my excruciating defecatory urge, unlike Emanuele, who usually rushes to the toilet as soon as these embarrassing symptoms occur.

I start to repeat in my mind, like a mantra or a prayer, the words *seduta analitica – seduta analitica*. This Italian term means 'analytic session' but can also be interpreted as 'analytic seated'. Meanwhile the similarity of the word 'analytic' to 'anal-ytic' dawns on me. I continue to mentally repeat *seduta anal-itica!*, as if I was giving myself a command, as one would with an unruly dog. I intuitively feel that these words are crucially important, and that if I maintain my faith in the 'anal-ytic process' it will help me to endure the agony. With difficulty I finally manage to expel the utterance, 'I can imagine how painful it is'. Emanuele then starts to tremble violently, as if in terror. In broken tones he says:

> I think that I felt very lonely when I was a child ... and even now I often feel lonely. My father was too intrusive. My mother was so cold. Because of all this when I'm afraid – of girls for example – I lock myself in the toilet, so I can be alone. I realize that when I'm scared or in pain I close myself off, and don't think about my problems anymore. But the less I think about them, the less I can deal with them. Look! I'm really shaking!

As soon as Emanuele finishes talking, the pain in my belly starts to disappear. A shiver of relief runs down my spine followed by a pleasant feeling of warmth and relaxation that slowly expands throughout my body. The spasms of anal pain I had suffered were similar to the *proctalgia fugax* that Richard Carvalho describes (2014, p. 374), in the form of a 'fleeting rectal pain' shortly before a psychoanalytic session, which he later found out corresponded to what his patient had experienced earlier that morning. Carvalho points out that the patient's sense of abandonment by a mother who had 'grossly neglected' her was so painful that it couldn't be thought of and could only be manifested and communicated via a somatic symptom.

In much the same way that Carvalho and his patient shared the same dissociated symptom, which they were then gradually able to elaborate, also between Emanuele and myself a crucial event of deep *Coniunctio* had taken place in the third area, involving the healing of his mind/body splitting and allowing us to gain access to the structuring energy of the Self. My pain in the anus allowed me to gain an embodied awareness of Emanuele's separation anxiety, which had triggered off the aggressive and omnipotent fantasy of possessing the mother-analyst, in order to negate her-his absence. At the beginning of therapy Emanuele saw me as a father and 'anal/genital intruder' (Clark, 1996, p. 361), who invaded his private sphere by means of interpretations. But then, after his defences had been eroded, I became a mother-analyst whose intolerable absences (for example over the Christmas holiday) triggered off erotic fantasies of incorporation and possession. There was thus an attempt to transform the analytical relationship into an 'anal relationship' of retention and control, and to annul the suffering of separation through the omnipotent fantasy of 'possessing' the analyst.

At such crucial moments of analysis the patient's intolerable affects can remain blocked within the analyst's body in the form of unelaborated somatic symptoms, which can sometimes lead to genuine health problems (Addison, 2019, p. 87; Corsa and Monterosa, 2015, p. 83; Redfearn, 2000, p. 182). Godsil (2018, p. 9) explains how the psychic contagion can remain 'mute' and latent within the analyst's body as a somatic residue caused by a psychotic absence of differentiation unconsciously induced by the patient.

Over the course of analysis Emanuele and I entered a psychoid realm in which 'concern over which parts of the psyche belong to whom fades' (Schwartz-Salant, 1989, p. 109). Here, while sharing our bodily sensations, we could connect with the life-giving forces of the collective unconscious. Our painful but fruitful analytical relationship, with its complexual as well as more broadly archetypal dynamics, had made it possible for him to move from an omnipotent attempt to carnally possess his analyst to finally obtaining symbolic possession of an internal analyst who could reactivate his process of individuation and safeguard its continued vigour and transformative activity in future.

According to Mara Sidoli, omnipotence – employed as a defence against separation anxiety and as an attempt to control processes of deintegration/reintrojection that are experienced as catastrophic – recedes at the very moment in which the archetypal images 'become incarnated in human experiences' providing the individual with 'a sense of realistic limitations' (Sidoli, 2000, p. 36).

In fact from this moment on Emanuele began to develop a greater sense of adequacy and self-sufficiency and to attain significant personal and professional goals. He started to have a stable relationship with a girl of his own age and successfully applied for a job with an excellent salary. Finally he found the courage to leave the family home and went to live with a friend in rented accommodation.

Conclusions

In this chapter I have attempted to identify the main aspects of the phenomenon of unconscious somatic communication, applying the Jungian hypothesis of a somato-psychic area shared by the patient and analyst. I have illustrated how affects connected with preverbal experiences of unthinkable psychic pain can manifest in the patient's body as somatic disturbances caused by the defence mechanism of mind/body splitting, compounded by the difficulty or impossibility of mentally representing intolerable affects. These can then break into the analyst's body, by means of the mechanism of projective identification that summons the analyst to work upon his/her own somatic experiences produced by contact with the split-off complexes of the analysand.

The lack of boundaries within the analytic dyad can be disorienting and confusing, but this is what makes it possible to directly get in touch with the patient's dissociative defensive mechanisms and experience the patient's embodied suffering. As analysts, we must 'bear what is felt to be unbearable' (Cavalli, 2020, p. 789) and tolerate the 'sense of confusion, mourning over our inability to figure things out, our sense of failure or uncertainty, before we can help the patient work through similar anxiety.' (Waska, 2014, p.101).

We then need to work with our somatic symptoms, transforming them by means of an embodied *rêverie*, which can merge these concrete manifestations with images that spontaneously arise in the analyst's mind, conjured up by the split-off psychic contents of the analysand, who can then gradually be led to a new relational bond through the analyst's containment, sympathy and understanding. This experience mends and heals the patient's mind/body splitting, leading to a psychosomatic partnership, by means of which s/he can perceive and progressively elaborate his/her inner psychic pain. The 'restoration of the body-mind connection' (Wright, 2020, p. 553) within the analytical relationship permits the reconciliation and reconjunction of mind and matter, the two poles of the archetype of the Self.

The analytic dyad can now move from a complexual personal level to an archetypal and collective level, and enter a shared unconscious realm in which the self-healing vivifying energies of the collective unconscious can reactivate the patient's process of individuation. By sharing their experiences within this third area, the patient and the analyst influence and transform each other with profound and creative modalities that go beyond the restricted level of conscious understanding and rational discernment.

In fact, in this case, our experiences in analysis furthered not only Emanuele's process of individuation, but also my own, as I feel that it encouraged me to embark upon an exciting and inspiring journey of personal maturation and professional growth. I became involved in several stimulating and rewarding initiatives regarding the role of the body in analysis, including the participation in several conferences, leading to the writing of this chapter. Starting from an intense analytic experience I have become involved in a field of collective research that has been developing in some very interesting ways and that has allowed me to have many fruitful encounters with analysts and researchers, in Italy as well as abroad.

NOTE TO THE READER

This chapter is based on a prior publication of the author, 'Embodying analysis: the body and the therapeutic process' (2016). He gratefully acknowledges permission from the Journal of Analytical Psychology *to reprint this previously published material.*

In addition, I wish to express my gratitude to my translator, Mr Tristam Bruce, for his excellent work and useful feedback.

CHAPTER 7

Revisiting the entropic body: when the body is the canvas

Tom Wooldridge

Introduction

In a previous paper (Wooldridge, 2018), I developed the notion of *the entropic* body: a false body (Orbach, 1986, 2002, 2009; Goldberg, 2004) employed by patients with anorexia nervosa in an attempt to compensate for the failure to internalize maternal comforting functions that could transform catastrophic anxiety into signal anxiety. This body-state (Petrucelli, 2015) develops against a background of profound early trauma in which the environment has repeatedly failed to regulate the child's anxiety, leaving her unable to regulate her own anxiety or to turn to others for help in doing so. This chapter explores the way in which the entropic body serves to communicate, albeit not in symbolic form, this early traumatic experience and the catastrophic anxiety patients are attempting to regulate through their omnipotent defences. Unable to relate to their anxiety as a signal and with their symbolic capacity impaired, patients with anorexia nervosa instead express in concrete form the complex affects with which they struggle on the canvas of their own bodies.

Anorexia nervosa consists of a restriction of energy intake leading to a significantly low body weight and an intense fear of becoming fat (American Psychiatric Association, 2013). A review of nearly 50 years of research confirms that it has the highest mortality rate of any mental illness (Arcelus et al., 2011). Adolescents and young adults with anorexia nervosa have ten times the risk of dying compared to their same-aged peers (Smink, Hoeken and Hoek, 2012). According to Steinhausen (2009), only 46 per cent of patients fully recover from anorexia nervosa, a third improve with only partial or residual features and 20 per cent remain chronically ill from the long term. Men and boys represent 25 per cent of individuals with anorexia nervosa and are at a higher risk of dying (Mond, Mitchinson and Hay, 2014), in part because they are often diagnosed later because eating disorders are often thought of as a 'female problem' (Wooldridge, 2016; Wooldridge and Lytle, 2012). With anorexia nervosa having the highest mortality rate of any psychiatric disorder, weight restoration is the foremost treatment priority. The 'gold standard' treatment for patients in this stage is family-based therapy (FBT), which promotes an 'agnostic' position with regard to aetiological factors, particularly the family's role in the child's developing an eating disorder (Lock and Le Grange, 2015). As I stated in a previous article (Wooldridge, 2018), this reflects a larger trend in which real engagement with the patient's illness and underlying psychic pain is neglected in favour of rapid symptom reduction, driven by numerous factors including the anxiety of treatment providers as well as institutional and economic imperatives. Because treatment for anorexia nervosa is now highly medicalized, the patient's subjectivity is often forgotten (Wooldridge, 2018).

Family-based therapy and related treatments have a strong track record at mitigating shame and stigma so that young people with anorexia nervosa can engage in treatment oriented toward weight restoration. In fact, I often refer my adolescent patients to providers who offer this form of treatment. In a previous book, I advocated for the importance of treatment teams (Wooldridge, 2016). As part of such a treatment team, I believe that psychoanalytic and other depth-based treatments also have an important role to play, because even when weight restoration has been achieved, the underlying intrapsychic dynamics that contributed to the development of the eating disorder are typically still in place and, equally important, all patients need a space in which the emotional truth of their experience can be acknowledged and thought about as fully as possible.

There is a substantial literature on eating disorders within the psychoanalytic tradition. Although it appears that Freud did not treat patients with eating disorders, there are numerous references to eating disturbances in his writings (Caparrotta and Ghaffari, 2006). Early on, drive theorists linked anorexia nervosa to problems in the oral phase of psychosexual development, describing the punitive superego and self-denial that accompanied these patients' normal oral impulses. In this paradigm, self-starvation was often understood as a defence against fantasies of oral impregnation (Moulton, 1942; Rowland, 1970; Waller, Kaufman and Deutsch, 1940).

Much more widely recognized, Bruch's (1962, 1973, 1978) writings, which also reached the lay public, described anorexia nervosa in the language of object relations. Self-starvation was cast as a struggle for autonomy, mastery and self-esteem. In her view, disruptions in the early mother–child relationship make the child vulnerable to developing the disorder during adolescence: a time that demands a greater ability for autonomous functioning in the adolescent. Self psychologists have described developmental failures in the processes of mirroring and idealization that contribute to vulnerabilities in self-esteem and self-cohesion. From this perspective, eating disorders serve restorative and regulatory functions for the self. Patients with anorexia nervosa are seen as presenting a facade of pseudo-self-sufficiency in the face of parents who are self-absorbed, anxious or emotionally impermeable (Goodsitt, 1997).

Over the past decade, there has been a developing interest in the role of trauma and dissociation in eating disorders. From this perspective, eating disorder symptoms hold dissociated parts of the patient's self and relational history (Petrucelli, 2015). Starvation, bingeing and purging, for example, are understood as dissociative processes and, as such, are attempts to maintain self-continuity and self-organization. As part of this emerging literature, Petrucelli (2015), drawing on Bromberg's (1998, 2006, 2011) vision of the self as dissociatively organized into self-states by pervasive relational trauma, developed the notion of *body states*. Much of our affect does not yet exist in representational form – as words and images – but instead lives in the body, upon and through which that affect is expressed. For patients with eating disorders, body states hold affect-laden 'material' ripe for elaboration by the analyst and patient, who make up an intersubjectively communicating – body state to body state – dyad. This dyad is what makes it possible to gain enough purchase outside a particular body state to begin to elaborate it in this way. Of particular interest in this elaboration are the relational meanings of the patient's body states, both as they emerged in early development and manifest now, in the analytic couple.

The present chapter[1] revisits my own notion of the entropic body as the body state that characterizes anorexia nervosa.[2] In doing so, I will highlight – consistent with the theme of this book – how the entropic body communicates important aspects of the patient's emotional experience, both in the present and in childhood, though this emotional experience cannot (yet) be rendered in words and images. The traumatic themes (Shabad, 1993; Wooldridge, in press b) – one of which is described below – that contribute to anorexia nervosa, because they are traumatic, hobble the mind's ability to represent and symbolize (Lecours and Bouchard, 1997) the affects they evoke, which accounts for the fact that patients with anorexia nervosa are frequently described as alexithymic (Westwood et al., 2017). Unable to convey in words and images the emotional pain that drives their eating disorder, the patient's body becomes the canvas that, over time, must be 'decoded' by patient and analysts so that its meaning can be fully understood.

Anorexia nervosa and traumatic themes

Over the past several years, I have written a series of articles that elaborate my own perspectives on anorexia nervosa (Wooldridge, 2014, 2016, 2018, submitted, in press a, in press b). In my clinical experience, in many patients with anorexia nervosa, analytic inquiry suggests a particular kind of breakdown in containment in early life (Bion, 1962) in which mother uses her child as a receptacle for her own unprocessed anxieties and affects. This traumatic theme (Shabad, 1993) leads to the development of a 'no-entry system of defence' (Williams, 1997) that covers over their experience of having been permeable in this way. This system consists of a defensive rejection of input not confined to food intake but manifesting across the patient's character. In this vein, Zerbe (1993) observes that the refusal of food is 'an autonomous statement, par excellence: 'I don't need you. I don't need anything. I don't even need food to survive. I am totally independent" (p. 95). Chasseguet-Smirgel (1993, 1995), similarly, suggests that anorexic patients attempt on the level of unconscious fantasy to function in an autarchical manner, without need of nourishment, literal and figurative, from external sources, especially the primary object.

In a previous series of articles (Wooldridge, 2018, 2014), I discussed the case of 'Sara', a woman in her late teens with anorexia nervosa who I saw for nearly a decade in psychoanalytic psychotherapy.[3] Born six weeks premature, her family was uncertain for several weeks whether she would live and for a substantial period of time, she was only kept alive inside an incubator, isolated from human contact. Her childhood was filled with innumerable visits to the doctor, described by her as both emotionally and physically intrusive, and the narrative of her early family life also included many instances of feeling emotionally invaded by her parents. Similarly, in the early period of our work together, my comments were experienced by her as 'piercing' and 'penetrating'. This, we came to understand, was connected to her rejection of food: above all, she wanted to keep what was outside her, experienced as dangerous, outside where it belonged.

As I described previously (Wooldridge, 2018), work on this traumatic theme may reveal a developmentally more primitive set of difficulties. Experiences of overwhelming affect, whether in isolation or as the cumulative trauma of the caretaker's repeated failure over time to serve as a shield (Khan, 1963), disorganize the ego and threaten its cohesion and differentiation. This undermines the development of signal anxiety and associated higher-order capacities to provide oneself comfort and to seek comfort from others. Consider the following excerpt:

Sara: I tried walking here more slowly today. Without the music, the audio books I usually listen to. You were right, it was hard.

Analyst: What came up for you?

Sara: It's hard to describe. I kept saying to myself, in my internal monologue, you know, 'There's a pain that shatters.' It's like I'm remembering, but I don't know what I'm remembering.

Analyst: That's something you've known before, shattering.

Sara: Yes, and that's what it feels like when I'm fighting with my mom, too, that I'm going to fall apart if she leaves, or even when she walks into the other room during a fight, leaving me by myself.

Analyst: That's the anxiety we've been talking about, that fear of falling apart in some way.

In this excerpt, Sara describes her experience of affective overwhelm that, it seems to her, threatens the integrity of her mind. In the face of this unbearable tension, patients with anorexia nervosa emaciate their bodies to create a second skin (Bick, 1968) as a substitute for these higher-order capacities. The progression that I observe in patients takes the following form: first, the anxieties began to manifest as the fear and the feeling of becoming fat – of falling apart, a mess of loose skin, bulging stomach, flabby arms. Then caloric restriction counters this experience and leads to the feeling of being lean and compact – in essence, together once more. The experience of starvation – the intensity of its sensations – forms a physical shell that replaces the holding ordinarily provided by human relationship, whether with caretaker or analyst. This shell is the body state that I referred to as the entropic body, a form of the false body.[4]

Signal anxiety and annihilation anxiety

In previous articles, I have suggested that trauma lies at the core of many (though perhaps not all) cases of anorexia nervosa (Wooldridge, 2018, in press b). In speaking of trauma, I am referring to experiences that exceed the individual's capacity for emotional self-regulation and for representing and symbolizing emotional experience so that it can be reflected upon (see Brown, 2019 for a fuller treatment of psychoanalytic thinking about trauma). This, in turn, leads to a traumatic organization characterized by cognitive concreteness – the eating disorder and its associated alexithymia – that holds and repetitively enacts the underlying affects in a desperate attempt to work through the relevant traumatic themes but which actually traps the patient more deeply in them. Although different traumatic themes contribute to anorexia nervosa in different patients, I have previously suggested that in many cases of anorexia nervosa, experiences of overwhelming affect, whether in isolation or as the cumulative trauma of the caretaker's repeated failure over time to serve as a shield (Khan, 1963), threatened the integrity of the ego. This, in turn, undermines the development of signal anxiety and associated higher-order capacities to provide oneself comfort and to seek comfort from others. In the face of this, the anorexic patient must search for other means to contend with overwhelming annihilation anxiety.[5]

Later in analysis, Sara recounted almost daily fights with her mother.

After each, she would think to herself, 'She's done with me,' and the following day at school would be filled with terror that her mother wouldn't be there when she arrived home afterwards. This terror, which we came to call the experience of falling forever (Winnicott, 1974) in which there would be no one she could rely upon for an emotional floor, was still very much alive for her as an adolescent and drove her to starve herself as her best attempt at comforting herself in the face of it. It was not until several years into treatment, however, that we could begin to understand the meaning of this terror, which until then was experienced as meaningless. Over time, Sara developed the capacity to make use of her anxiety as a signal of the need to seek comfort from her analyst and later, from others.

Sara: Last night I was on the phone with my mother and she was so angry with me. I tried to speak up, to ask her to calm down, and that only made her even more angry. Finally, she slammed down the phone without saying goodbye. It was like being whipped around in a whirlwind. I have been so anxious since that happened.

Analyst: Can you say more about the anxiety?

Sara: My heart is racing ... my stomach hurts ... it's like I'm tensing my whole body against it.

Analyst: You can feel it in your body – this anxiety – but it's harder to get a hold of the feelings that go with it. You might feel afraid she'll hold a grudge for a long time or, even worse, never talk with you again. Like you worried she might do when you were little.

Sara: That's it! I always feel better when we seem to make up later. You know, I had the impulse to call you last night ... I didn't do it, ultimately, but I thought about it. Just thinking about it actually made me feel better. I remember thinking, 'I'm upset that she's going to get rid of me.' It took me a while to get to that, but I did, and then I thought of you.

In healthy development, anxiety begins to serve as a signal (Freud, 1926) through repeated interactions between mother and infant, and later between the child and her larger environment. If these interactions are 'good enough', the child internalizes the environment's soothing functions. Pine (1983) provides a compelling description of this situation: the human is born helpless in the face of mounting tensions until the mother arrives or defensive manoeuvres (i.e. dissociative mechanisms such as apathy or sleep) are employed. From this state of boundless tension, a higher order anxiety, which serves as a signal to trigger psychological manoeuvres to regulate tension, evolves in the course of healthy development. Pine (1983) describes this as follows:

> The infant who has been reliably gratified when hungry, for example, can gradually come to greet a new occasion of hunger differently from one who has not been so gratified. The memory of repeated pairings of hunger and satisfaction sets up an anticipation that satisfaction will again be forthcoming, an anticipation that by another name we call basic trust. In that moment of delay, when the anticipation of gratification (or the recognition of danger and the memory of its prior resolution) slows the rate of development of tension, higher order adaptive behaviour (calling mother), or, later, intrapsychic defences (withdrawal of interest from the psychological danger situation, averting one's thoughts, stifling the affect), come into play. This occurs rather than having the first sign of anxiety, in snowballing fashion, stimulate the memory of previous panic, thus leading rapidly to an escalation of the anxiety once again to panic proportions (p. 244).

Signal anxiety is a necessary ingredient in an individual's capacity to communicate his distress both to himself and to the people in his environment. It is fundamental to our ability to trust (Erikson, 1993) that others will hear our calls of distress and that communicating that distress to them will bring relief. But what happens if the development of signal anxiety has been disrupted, leaving the organism flooded with anxiety that cannot be organized through higher-order capacities? The anorexic patient seeks a way to attenuate emotional pain and the entropic body provides one such means of doing so. In lieu of communication with another person, the body becomes the canvas upon and through which this intolerable agony (Winnicott, 1974) is conveyed.

In this vein, consider the following memory that Sara recounted in our work together:

Sara: When I was young – maybe two or three – I'd call out in the night because I was upset. But I didn't scream for my mother or father. I'd wake up at 2 a.m. and yell, 'Cookie! Cookie!' I've never been able to understand that, why I didn't want my mother or my father. The only source of comfort I could imagine was a cookie.

We came to believe that in asking for a cookie, Sara was not, as some children might be, asking for comfort from her parents; rather, she was simply asking for a cookie. She had, I believe, given up most of her hope that relationships could provide comfort. The only comfort that could be imagined was from a concrete object – notably, given her later eating disorder, from food. Because this was an inadequate solution, her anxiety escalated into almost perpetual terror: a terror that she could not name or understand but that was threaded through nearly every moment of her life.

The entropic body

When I first used the term *entropic body* (Wooldridge, 2018), I was poetically referring to Freud's (1920) conception of the death drive as aiming toward a state that can be described with words like tension reduction, dedifferentiation, unbinding and dissolution. As I wrote, 'Patients with anorexia nervosa emaciate their bodies to create an experience of somatic entropy – that is, stasis and tension reduction' (Wooldridge, 2018, p. 199). Setting aside Freud's (1920) speculations about the biological basis of the death drive, I was interested in the phenomenological sphere he was describing. I understood the patients with anorexia nervosa as moving toward this sphere in an effort to survive the failure to internalize anxiety-regulating, soothing functions in early development and to dissociate a profound yearning for anxiety-regulating contact with another person.

The idea of the entropic body first occurred to me when I noticed Winnicott's (1974) brief comment that the fear of falling forever – one of his ways of describing the phenomenological experience of intolerable agony resulting from infantile trauma – is defended against by 'self-holding' (p.

104). Bick (1968), it occurred to me, evocatively describes one form this self-holding might take in her article on second-skin formations. In her view, patients may engage physical and muscular capacities to constitute a 'second skin' in lieu of the function that ought to be provided by a containing object in early development which, over time, would facilitate the actual skin functioning as a boundary between inside and outside and holding the self together.

The entropic body takes the following form: first, the anxieties began to manifest as the terror and subjective experience of becoming fat – of falling apart, a mess of loose skin, bulging stomach, flabby arms. Then caloric restriction counters this experience and leads to the feeling of being lean and compact – in short, together once more. The experience of starvation – the intensity of its physical and emotional sensations – forms a physical shell that replaces the holding ordinarily provided by human relationship, whether with caretaker or analyst. This shell is the body state that I call the entropic body, which provides a primitive form of self-holding in the face of intolerable annihilation anxiety that cannot be regulated within the self or in contact with another person. At the time, I attempted to describe the experience of the entropic body as follows:

> Imagine the starving body. The hands and feet are frightfully cold and numb. The stomach and cheeks are concave, sunken in on themselves, and the protrusions of the ribs painful against the thin and brittle skin. Not only is this startling to outside observers, but these physical changes are also palpable for patients themselves. Many of my patients report being able to feel their heartbeat even when they are physically at rest. A sort of deadening calm descends upon mind and body, flattening out all signs of living vitality. The ring of desire can only be heard in the far away distance. Indeed, it has often been pointed out that significant weight loss elicits physiological adaptations that reduce arousal. With prolonged starvation, parasympathetic activation is increased (Miller, Redlich and Steiner, 2003) and bradycardia often develops (Mitchell and Crow, 2006). These physiological adaptations reduce the overall intensity of affect (Craig, 2004) and also mute hunger cues (Wang, Hung and Randall, 2006) (Wooldridge, 2018, p. 198).

Bick (1968), in her article, notes that this phenomenon can be seen in the transference in the context of dependence and separation. In our work together, Sara was increasingly able to make use of the holding our relationship provided to bear the intensity of her anxieties about falling apart without resorting to self-starvation. In our relationship she had found a way to communicate in words and images about the intolerable agony of both her early and present experience. Before an extended vacation in the early period of analysis, however, she began to increase her food restriction once again. My vacation forced her to confront her dependence upon me, which resonated with past experiences of being left without emotional contact. Because she could not communicate with me during my vacation both concretely and internally (she could not yet 'hold on' to me during my absence), she again turned to self-starvation as an omnipotent means of managing overwhelming anxieties while also dissociating the pains of separation and loss associated with dependence upon me. Her body again became the canvas upon and through which her pain was conveyed.

The body as canvas: the role of alexithymia

After developing the notion of the entropic body (Wooldridge, 2018), I became interested in the prevalence of alexithymia in patients with anorexia nervosa (Wooldridge, in press b). As described above, in many cases of anorexia nervosa analytic inquiry reveals the presence of a particular kind of breakdown of containment in early life (Bion, 1962) in which mother uses her child as a receptacle for her own unprocessed anxieties and affects (Williams, 1997). This traumatic theme (Shabad, 1993) impairs the mind's ability to symbolize and represent the affects it evokes and thus significantly contributes to the alexithymia frequently observed in patients with anorexia nervosa.

When Sara began treatment with me, she knew that she was anxious and, relatively quickly, was able to understand that her self-starvation provided relief from that anxiety. She was not, however, able to put into words *why* she felt so terrified. It was only through several years of analytic work, in which I made quite active use of my own symbolic capacities, that she was able to begin to develop a narrative that felt adequate to the intensity of her feelings. This narrative emerged from the work that we did together to elaborate her experience into images and words.

Coined by Sifneos (1973), alexithymia comes from the Greek (a = lack, lexis = word, thymus = emotion) and refers to a cluster of features including difficulty identifying and describing subjective feelings, a circumscribed fantasy life and an externally oriented thinking style (Taylor and Bagby, 2013). Upon its introduction as a formal construct, it was of interest to psychoanalysts engaged in the treatment of psychosomatic diseases and, shortly thereafter, was incorporated into the wider field of research on emotional processing and affect pathology (Taylor and Bagby, 2013). It has been noted in patients with post-traumatic states (Krystal, 1968), drug dependence (Krystal and Raskin, 1970), eating disorders (Bruch, 1971, 1973, 1978) and panic disorder (Nemiah, 1984). This is consistent with the idea that emotion, unsymbolized, can generate bodily symptoms secondary to unregulated activation of visceral/motoric systems (Taylor and Bagby, 2013).[6]

Empirical research has established that alexithymia co-occurs with eating disorders of all subtypes (Westwood et al., 2017) and with eating disorder symptomatology that does not rise to the level of a diagnosis (e.g. Ridout et al., 2010; De Berardis et al., 2007). Whereas some studies have reported no significant differences in alexithymia across eating disorder diagnoses, others have suggested that individuals with anorexia nervosa experience higher levels (Nowakowski, McFarlane and Cassin, 2013). Alexithymia appears to decrease significantly post-treatment with all eating disorders (Nowakowski, McFarlane and Cassin, 2013). Increasingly, evidence suggests correlations between alexithymia and insecure attachment (Scheidt et al., 1999; De Rick and Vanheule, 2006; Montebarocci et al., 2004; Troisi et al., 2001) and psychic trauma (Krystal, 1968). Several studies have shown that alexithymia is associated with retrospectively reported experiences of emotional and/or physical neglect or childhood sexual or physical abuse (Berenbaum, 1996; Frewen et al., 2008; Paivio and McCulloch, 2004; Zlotnick, Mattia and Zimmerman, 2001). Other empirical studies have linked alexithymia to trauma in adulthood (Frewen et al., 2008; Taylor, 2004).

There is now a significant literature on unrepresented states of mind: mental contents not stored in symbolic form as words or images (e.g. Bion, 1962; Green, 1975; Matte-Blanco, 1988; Lecours and Bouchard, 1997; Botella and Botella, 2005). The concept of alexithymia emerged as the field was starting to theorize these unrepresented states and groups together patients for whom the capacity to symbolize affect is significantly impaired. Nemiah (1977) aptly described the underdeveloped capacity in alexithymic patients: *the psychic elaboration of emotion*, through which emotions come to be represented mentally and experienced as feelings. This has been termed the 'immune system of the psyche', for it absorbs external stresses as well as internal pressures by mentally processing their effects on the body and elaborating them further (Lecours and Bouchard, 1997). The successful treatment of anorexia nervosa entails the development of this capacity so that the body no longer is the primary vehicle through and upon which these affects can be communicated. With this capacity intact, the patient can begin to use words to express the profound emotional distress that has given rise to, and continues to drive, her eating disorder. Of course, the capacity for the psychic elaboration of emotion, as Bion (1962) so eloquently described, develops through relationship.

It is important to highlight the slow, painstaking work that was required for Sara and I to collaboratively develop her capacity to represent and symbolize (Lecours and Bouchard, 1997) her emotional experience. At times, I attempted to put words to her distress too quickly, which unfortunately recreated the experience of being penetrated and pierced by something dangerous outside of herself. Each time this happened, a period of emotional repair, which was quite trying for us both, was required and I sought to more accurately attune myself to what she could and could not tolerate thinking about. At other times, I also struggled to find words for her experience; the horror of some of her memories was too much for me to encompass. Nonetheless, after several years of work together, her capacity for the psychic elaboration of emotion (Nemiah, 1977) was far more developed. What she was once only able to describe in concrete, impoverished terms, she is now able to put into complex, multi-faceted descriptions that do justice to her experience and provide a way to 'bind' the painful feelings that are part of that experience.

Conclusions

For many patients with anorexia nervosa, analytic inquiry suggests a particular kind of breakdown in containment in early life (Bion, 1962) in which mother uses her child as a receptacle for her own unprocessed anxieties and affects. This traumatic theme (Shabad, 1993) leads to the development of a 'no-entry system of defense' (Williams, 1997) that covers over their experience of having been permeable in this way. Work on this traumatic theme may reveal a developmentally more primitive set of difficulties: experiences of overwhelming affect, whether in isolation or as the cumulative trauma of the caretaker's repeated failure over time to serve as a shield (Khan, 1963), disorganize the ego and threaten its cohesion and differentiation. This undermines the development of signal anxiety and associated higher-order capacities to provide oneself comfort and to seek comfort from others. It also disrupts the development of the patient's developing symbolic capacity and contributes to the alexithymia that is associated with anorexia nervosa. With the capacity for signal anxiety disrupted, the patient is flooded with anxiety that cannot be organized through higher-order capacities and seeks a way to attenuate emotional pain. The entropic body provides one such means of doing so. In lieu of communication with another person, the body becomes the canvas upon and through which this intolerable agony (Winnicott, 1974) is conveyed.

Notes

1. An important limitation of the present chapter is that it does not incorporate the vast literature on sociocultural factors that contribute to eating disorders. Because of space limitations, I am not able to do justice to the many important contributions that have been made, including research on the idealization of the thin body type within Western society (Bruch, 1962; Garner et al., 1980), the role of the mass media in promoting pathogenic attitudes toward the body and self (Stice et al., 1994), the promotion of dieting behaviour in athletes such as ballerinas, models, jockeys and wrestlers (Garner and Garfinkel, 1980; Mickalide, 1990; Wooldridge, 2016; Wooldridge and Lytle, 2012), and the influence of ethnic group values upon the development and experience of eating disorders (George and Franko, 2010).
2. As a descriptive diagnosis, anorexia nervosa does not refer to a single structural entity and, thus, any theoretical formulation of the disorder will be more or less applicable to an individual

patient. The perspective outlined here describes the dynamics of a variant of anorexia nervosa commonly encountered in clinical practice.
3. Identifying information has been altered to protect the patient's confidentiality.
4. Goldberg (2004) describes how some patients use their bodies to achieve emotional security through dissociation from bodily vitality, experienced as intolerable. Through a regime of psychosomatic control and auto-stimulation, the body is forced to react 'on cue' in order to contrive a predictable false vitality so that, over time, the natural rhythms of the body are brought under omnipotent control and replaced by coerced forms of bodily aliveness. This somatic false self creates a buffer against both external impingement and internal objects, which are felt to threaten the self with fragmentation. This strategy leads to an experience of mastery and orients the self toward social adaptation but also dissociates underlying vitality, desire and need and leaves the self vulnerable to the threat of meaninglessness.
5. Both Freud (1926) and Winnicott (1974) provide evocative ways of describing the phenomenological experience of annihilation anxiety. Freud (1926) describes a sequence of 'danger situations' that he imagined might feel like threats to the structure and integrity of the self. These include overwhelming excitation, the loss of the object, the loss of the object's love, and castration anxiety. In more evocative language, Winnicott (1974) lists a number of forms this anxiety can take, including a return to an unintegrated state, falling forever, loss of psychosomatic collusion, loss of sense of the real, and loss of capacity to relate to objects.
6. As Taylor and Bagby (2013) point out, alexithymia is a dimensional construct instead of an all-or-none phenomenon.

CHAPTER 8

When the psyche shreds and the body takes over

William F. Cornell

When I sit to begin writing, I locate myself in one of two places. The first is my study. Over my desk are images of Bob Dylan and Johnny Cash, to my left a wall of books, and to my right photographs of my family and a painting by my partner, Mick. When I am surrounded by working books and texts too numerous for my desk, I move to the dining room table where I face photos of my grandsons, artwork by Mick and local artists, and my CD collection. Bach or Philip Glass are typically playing – loud if I am alone in the house. It is within this deeply sensate, non-verbal environment that I begin to find my words and my thinking gradually becomes structured. I am reminded, too, of the first time I met Danielle Quinodoz (2003) whose writing had often informed and inspired me. She offered to show me her office. I had known her then only as a neo-Kleinian analyst, so the office I imagined for her was quite severe, impersonal. Instead, I walked into a warm, deeply personal room full of objects that conveyed a sense of age and personal associations. She explained that nearly everything in her office had some connection to her parents and grandparents, telling me the history of each. When I expressed surprise that her office setting was so personal, Danielle replied, 'We can only do this work when we are surrounded by objects of those we love and who loved us.' Danielle was not speaking of her internal objects, but of the concrete, visible, touchable objects that evoked her rich internal world and enlivened her working environment.

The verbal and symbolic order had come to be the primary means and vocabulary of psychoanalytic treatment, but in recent decades there has been increasing recognition and exploration of the place of visual, sensate, motoric, and visceral modes of experience and expression within the analytic endeavour. The bodies of clients and therapists alike are now increasingly understood to be active, informative domains of the therapeutic field. As I approach what I hope to be able to convey in the essay – using the written word to attempt to convey unlanguaged experience – I wanted to situate the reader in the physicality of my working environment.

While one's physical, sensate world can represent and vitalize one's internal object world with a sense of memory, belonging and meaning, the sensate body may also – of self-protective necessity – come to defend against memory and meaning, replacing the people and experiences that have been threatening sources of chaos or annihilation. As Lombardi (2008) observes, 'We should not forget that, if the body can become the cradle of the processes of mental signification, it can also be their grave, if the relationship with the body "saturates" (Bion, 1970) instead of initiating development towards emotion and thought' (p. 394).

Having been originally trained as a neo-Reichian body psychotherapist (Cornell, 2015, 2009b) my practice has always had what may be a higher frequency of clients for whom their bodies have been a source of anxiety and disturbance. Over the years I have witnessed a spectrum of bodily based distresses, ranging from fabricated bodies (Goldberg, 2004; Yarom, 2015) that have more or less consciously constructed to ward off anxiety and shame, to those plagued by psychosomatic distress and obsessional preoccupations dissociated from both the vulnerabilities and vitalities of the body (Quinodoz, 2003; Aisenstein and de Aisemberg, 2010), and to those in which there is a psychotic level of splitting and disavowal between one's emotional/psychic life and that of the body (De Masi, 2009; Williams, 2010; Lombardi and Pola, 2010, Lombardi, 2016; Lombardi, Rinaldi and Thanopulos, 2019) or autistic encapsulations so vividly described by Tustin (1986), and Alvarez (1992, 2012).

With regard to 'primitive'

The term 'primitive' has come to be a common descriptor for these non-verbal, sensate dominated mental states and defences (Gedo, 1997; Ogden,

1989; Mitrani, 1996, 2007; Lombardi, 2002; Ferrari, 2004; Roussillon, 2011). The first dictionary definition of 'primitive' is that 'of or pertaining to the beginnings, the original state', followed by a second, 'characterized by simplicity, crudity, unsophisticated'. Given the psychoanalytic valorization of the verbal and symbolic, I see the application of that term 'primitive', unfortunately, too often conveying the second, rather than the first, meaning of the term. 'Primitive' can convey a derogatory tone with a diminishment and misrepresentation of psychic worlds of those whose lives and forms of communication are dominated by sensate experience and concrete objects, rather than verbal, symbolic language. Psychic maturation was marked in most psychoanalytic models by the development of the capacity for symbolic thinking. The 'primitive' has come to be equated with the infantile and pathological.

Caper's vision of the infant, informed by contemporary infant research, is quite different than Freud's: 'If we consider how much a normal infant learns in, say, the first two years of life, then its contact with reality compares favourably with that of any other stage of life' (1999, p. 71). It is important to note that much of this learning precedes the infant's development of language and symbolic thought. Caper addressed the equating of psychopathology with primitive mental states, arguing that 'by holding that ill adults have regressed to the state of mind of a normal infant or small child, we have confused destructive states of mind with normal ones (that is, ones containing the capacity for development)' (p. 78). In his brilliant study of *Vulnerability to Psychosis*, De Masi (2009) builds on Caper's perspective to conclude, 'In this author's view, a sick person was by no means the adult embodiment of a primitive mental state; instead, illness was the outcome of a state abnormal from the beginning' (p. 27). He goes on to argue, 'Whereas psychosis is a subversion of thought that leads to the disintegration of the mind, the magic world of the infant is open to the unknown and makes for the construction of personal meaning to be assigned to that world' (p. 30).

Furthermore, these sensory and motoric processes are not limited to infancy or crude, under-developed states of being. We do not grow out of these fundamental capacities as we mature. Quite the contrary, these are the vitalizing forces of life – indeed, the foundations of intimacy, play, eroticism, aggression, sexuality and nurturance throughout the course of life. Within the context of a reasonably responsible environment, this vital domain of experience forms the basis of a resonant and resilient sense of self. When the interpersonal/developmental environment is one of neglect or impingement/trauma, the capacity to integrate experience is diminished and the self learns to survive through varying degrees of dissociation, disavowal or psychotic splitting. Instead of 'primitive' I will be using adjectives such as foundational, essential, sensate and subsymbolic (Bucci, 2021) to convey the lived reality of sensation-defined modes of experience and expression.

Enlivening or deadening? The vital necessity of sensate/somatic organization

Ogden's (1989) vivid portrayal of what he termed the 'autistic-contiguous' mode of psychic organization opened a radically new understanding of deeply embedded, somatic structures for me. Ogden added 'contiguous' so as to provide a 'necessary antithesis to the connotations of isolation and disconnectedness carried by the word *autistic*' (p. 50, italics in original). While acknowledging the potential defensive functions of autistic encapsulation, Ogden also captures the vitality and function of sensate dominated modes of contact as 'the principal media for the creation of psychological meaning and the rudiments of the experience of self' (p. 52). Herein was again the dynamic, enlivening (rather than simply regressive) tension between protection and vitalizing.

Anzieu (1990, 2016) wrote a startling account of the functions of the skin in early psychological development, observing that 'the Skin-Ego arises in response to the need for a narcissistic wrapping and provides the psychical apparatus with a secure and consistent state of well-being' (2016, p. 43). Through the proprioceptive functions of the skin and the quality of skin to skin contact between parent and infant, the Skin-Ego provides the protocol, the felt and embodied means by which 'the Ego inherits the double faculty of setting up barriers (which become psychical defence mechanisms) and filtering exchanges (with the Id, the superego and the outside world). ... the Skin-Ego is the basis for the very possibility of thought' (2016, p. 44). Anzieu outlines the functions of the skin and Skin-Ego (pp. 103–18): holding, the incorporation of the parent's hands/ways of touching; containing; protection from noxious or invasive stimuli, individuation, i.e. the rudiments of selfhood; 'consensuality' (p. 112), which connects together sensations of differing kinds from different sources (internal and external); sexualization; libidinal recharging; and inscription, i.e. the registering of tactile, sensory traces.

The tactile, sensory modes of experience articulated by Ogden and Anzieu, while having infantile roots, remain vitalizing, organizing, libidinal forces throughout the course of life. These are essential both for self-organization (Cornell, 2008, 2011), the erotic forces of life and intimate, sexual relations over the course of life. Bucci (1997, 2021) has articulated (and through her decades of research into the psychotherapeutic process has *demonstrated*) a radically different understanding of 'primitive' modes of psychic organization and expression in her Multiple Code theory. She describes three modes of psychic organization and functioning – the verbal symbolic, non-verbal symbolic and subsymbolic – each of which is present through the course of life and which often need to become integrated through a referential process, which she sees as being at the heart of change through psychotherapy. She argues:

> Cognitive [and psychoanalytic] models have generally failed to consider the complexity and difficulty of the referential process. Standard views of cognitive development (Piaget, 1950; Bruner, 1966) have also failed to recognize the continuing role of nonverbal processing, including emotional information processing throughout life. In both of these developmental theories, it is assumed that earlier stages of concrete sensory and motoric processing drop out when levels of formal, logical processing are attained. These standard approaches to cognition must fail as the basis for a psychoanalytic theory ....
>
> Bucci (2021, p. 9)

The subsymbolic domains are seen through the Multiple Code theory as essential forms of psychic organization, means of *knowing* and *learning*, informing us about ourselves and others, consciously and unconsciously. There is vast potential for understanding and emotional contact when we open ourselves to *how* something is said and shown to us, as well as *how* we respond in pace, tone, postural shifts, facial expression, and so on. Multiple Code Theory provides a structure within which language/cognition and affect/body each have a place, a value and necessary functions through the interrelationship of three fundamental forms of psychic organization: verbal symbolic, non-verbal symbolic and subsymbolic.

Throughout this chapter I hope to convey the generative/communicative functions of unlanguaged experience as I also speak to the limiting and defensive consequences of sensate-dominated lives.

The adolescent body and the challenge of emergent sexuality

There has been a tendency within object relations models to attribute and explain severe psychopathologies anchored in the body as having been generated within chronic disturbances in the parent–infant relationships. There is, of course, an abundance of clinical evidence that can be viewed as supporting this emphasis. However, in my clinical experience, these disturbances are not limited to infancy but are all too often pervasive throughout a family system and over the course of a person's developmental stages. While I would certainly not minimize the long-term consequences of a distressed infancy, I am centred here on the chronic family, social and cultural environments that have attacked the individual's freedom and capacity to make meanings of their own lived experience, such that the sensate, physical world becomes a sanctuary and a primary, solitary source of safety, personal meaning and mental structure. Adolescence (Lombardi and Pola, 2010; Brady, 2016; Montemayor, 2019; Diem-Wille, 2021), as well as infancy, is a developmental crucible that is often catastrophic in its impact on a developing person's relationship to their own body and to the bodies of others. Lombardi and Pola (2010) address the impact of the adolescent body as the potential precipitant to psychotic levels of disorganization:

> Physical maturation at the same time confronts the [adolescent] subject with an *extraordinary intensification of the drives* and the real possibility of procreation. The body and the instincts make their presence urgently felt, thus fuelling a conflict that can assume psychotic proportions, with the consequent pressure to dissociate from the body as a source of containable turmoil.
> Lombardi and Pola (2010, p. 1420; italics in the original)

They stress:

> Given the overwhelming presence, in acute psychotic phases, of a sensory catastrophe ... the most urgent need is to provide first of all the spatio-temporal organization of bodily experience ... in other words, the elaborative resources of the analytic relationship should be directed towards confronting the manifestations of the most pressing 'object', which is, precisely, the body.
> Lombardi and Pola (2010, p. 1425)

The confrontation to which Lombardi and Pola refer is not so much that of the patient's body as that of the therapist. They stress the centrality of the therapist's access and use of their own somatic countertransference, such that 'it is *the totality of the analyst's person* that is involved, in the sense that the analyst is called upon to *contain first and foremost in his body* that presymbolic and concrete manifestations that "anticipate" the birth of emotional and mental phenomena' (p. 1425, italics in the original). The therapist's own somatic experience is seen here as essential to the treatment process as it is understood to be progressive rather than 'regressive' or defensive.

Our clinical and psychoanalytic literature all too often views lives lived with (and suffering from) obsessional/compulsive, psychosomatic and eating 'disorders' as the psychopathology of the individual, while we are immersed in a culture that idealizes the fabricated, unreal, phantasmic bodies of athletes who create machine-like bodies that continue to function at any cost, models (female and male) that 'grace' films, television and the covers of magazines, and the imagined bodies of pornography which can and will copulate with anyone and anything at any time. As Goldberg (2004) has observed in a compelling article describing the creation of 'fabricated bodies', 'Economic and cultural conditions furnish a variety of masks that may be adopted to provide the legitimacy for the fabrication of a well-regulated false body, and currently this appears most often to take place under the auspices of the ideology of health, self-improvement, and self-determination' (p. 824).

I now turn my attention to my therapeutic work with Sara, whose life was a decades-long struggle to differentiate herself from the catastrophe of a false body (Orbach, 1986, 2002, 2009), and a fabricated body

(Goldberg, 2004), forged in a fabricated family, so as to gradually establish a sense of personal identity and agency and her capacity for intimacy and adult sexuality. At the point when she sought psychotherapy, Sara's was a *viewed* body (Lemma, 2009; Cornell, 2019a) rather than a *lived* body. Given the severity and chronicity of Sara's somatic defences, analytic theories would likely suggest disturbances in the early mother/infant relations as the primary causal agents (Mitrani, 2007). But in Sara's we get a rather different picture, one that suggests that clinicians hold an open mind to the multiplicity of forces that can foster severe disturbances of one's relationship to one's own body.

Sara

As I began to think about possible case examples for this essay, I found it impossible to draw from work with current clients whose personal struggles are so highly individual that I could not find a way to accurately portray our work and adequately disguise their identities. So, I asked for the involvement of a former client, Sara, for whom I thought perhaps enough time had passed that we could talk, assess and write about our work with a bit more distance and reflectivity. She readily agreed, and then when we sat down in my office for the first time, she said, 'I read what you sent me. I really liked the way you described your study, your setting, the physical while you got ready to write. What you said about the body being seen as "primitive". What I understood you'd be writing about was how people used their bodies, how I used my body, to express what couldn't be expressed in any other fashion. Then after I agreed to do this my mind and my body both said NO! So, I talked with my husband. He thought this was an important invitation, and I decided to go ahead.' When I inquired as to how her body said 'NO,' Sara replied, 'Thinking about how my body says NO I realize it happens often, still. I feel cold in my belly sometimes even shiver, my focus goes out, my legs tighten ready to move, and I do move if I can (I suspect my over-exercising is to release frequent NO! episodes that I don't control by speaking or acting in a more direct manner).'

Sara and I worked together on and off for nearly 30 years, and over the course of that time my understanding and ways of working changed as much as Sara did. Our process of mutual learning should be evident in the unfolding of this clinical story. I interviewed Sara in my office to set the stage for my case discussion, portions of which are included here. As the article unfolded, I sent Sara drafts in an ongoing email dialogue that has further informed my reflections on our work together.

Sara was second born following a brother, who was named after his father. The first two years of her life seem to have been relatively peaceful. Her father was stationed away serving in the Army, so Sara, her mother and brother lived with their maternal grandparents. By the time she was three, her sister had been born and the family was now living on its own. Sara reports remembering great pleasure in helping take care of her little sister, and the violence and chaos of the family had not yet broken out. Sara recalls her mother taking her out of ballet lessons as a young girl telling her that if she continued, she would develop 'big thighs'. This was a harbinger of what was to come – a profound preoccupation from both parents on body image, on how she and they were seen by others and on 'perfection'.

My therapeutic work with Sara began in the 1970s, after I had been working with her schizophrenic brother, Larry, while she was still in high school. Larry (named after his father) had already been hospitalized three times with no significant improvement, and his daily life was one of dread, withdrawal or rage. Sara had been a part of family sessions that supplemented my work with her brother. I was director of a community mental health centre, that maintained an outpatient therapy clinic and also offered groups and classes in area schools and churches, all based in transactional analysis. After the family sessions, she enrolled in a 'TA for Teens' class and found, for the first time, a way to begin thinking about herself and her emotional struggles. Larry eventually left treatment with little improvement that I could see, although Sara reported in our interview that she did see improvement at home while he worked with me. He eventually moved out of state, living alone, and years later committed suicide.

The parents' position was that their son was the victim of flawed genes that were responsible for a history of mental illness through the family generations. It wasn't until years later, when I started working with Sara, that I learned that most of what I had been told while working with her brother were lies. Her brother and mother were both subject to violent rages from the father; that her mother became pregnant with Larry before marriage was another family secret.

Sara: I don't think my parents overtly recognized their own mental illness, my mother would call my father 'sick', but I think that referred to his addiction. She recognized Larry's mental illness and I don't think she ever admitted any responsibility or contribution. I think she thought he manifested the genes he inherited. She had a lot of shame I think from getting pregnant prior to marriage. When we were little, my mom was a great mom. She was a lot of fun when we were little kids. There was energy, humour, warmth when we were young. She did all sorts of creative things with us. We wrote a play. She made costumes. We practised. Tried to do it for Dad, and he just yelled, 'Get out of here!' Then as Dad got worse, she became like one of the kids, huddling with us in the corners. Hoping not to get screamed at. Larry would get beaten, and she did nothing. She had to save face in the neighbourhood, everywhere. She hid Larry's abuse, Dad's addiction. Once he cracked up the car. She covered it all up.

Sara's father had been a prominent local physician; he died when Sara was 10. Sara's mother had tried to escape her husband's rages and addiction by taking the family to live with her parents.

S: Mom's parents pushed her back to the marriage. She went partly because, apparently, he threatened to murder all of us including her parents. I remember my grandmother holding the phone saying to my mother, 'It's Larry, talk to him,' with this look and tone of complete admiration and saying words to the effect that he is changed.

Sara's mother and family returned to the father's home and continued violence. The public story was that he was so dedicated to his patients that he worked himself to death. The reality was that he was a self-prescribing drug addict who died of an overdose – whether intention or accidental was never clear, as that was covered up.

Bill: Your parents both being medical people. I've often wondered how that contributed to your preoccupation with your body, being clean, being 'healthy'.

S: I should have been a writer or a teacher, but I still had to prove myself that I could make it in Dad's field. I had no efficacy psychically to separate from her or him. There was no basement in my house. Fearful. It was an embarrassment to be ill. We were to have no needs. I fell off my bike and got gravel in my knees. I tried to fix it myself. My father had to do it. 'Stupid.' 'Shut up!', he shouted at me. He had to take me to his office to clean my knee. This was their work, and when they were home, no work. My father carried a large black medical bag with him everywhere, including syringes, which seemed normal to me as a kid (I occasionally raided the bag for dum-dum lollipops), but now I think he continually carried what he needed to dope himself. They also had a large metal storage cabinet in the garage that contained samples of any kind of medication a person might want. We used isopropyl alcohol and medical grade antibacterial cleansers. My father would take calls from patients at the dinner table. I knew way too much about things that could go wrong with the human body. I would hear these conversations and have a queasiness. I began to fear any symptom. I could feel others' bodies in my own.

After her father died, Sara's mother soon remarried, but her life did not improve. In fact, she found herself under ever increasing pressure to perform, succeed and fulfil the demands of a 'picture perfect' family.

S: After Dad died (Sara was 10), she married Elmer, and you know how that was. But still it was always, 'Sara, Sara, Sara, you have to do it.' When I left for college, I had no emotional resources. But I had to bring glory back to the family. It was such a burden. My first year in college was a triumph. I was an athlete. I became very popular. I was invited into sororities, the honour society. But I had diarrhoea, hives. I was exhausted. Sophomore year I tried to recreate that triumph. I failed. I switched schools. Decided to study nutrition. I had no support for an adult life, other than to bring home A's, the glory, and a husband.

I was so isolated. I did have two friends. They gave me bran muffins once, and I ate them all at once. Looking back, I can see that I was stuffing in all their nurturance. That's when the eating disorder switched and I became bulimic. I quit school. And I was eating, eating, eating.

Brady (2016) offers a series of compelling case studies in which she addresses adolescent struggles with eating disorders, cutting, substance abuse, suicidality and manic defences as varied manifestations of the bodily anguish and subsequent psychic isolation that threaten to tear an adolescent's life asunder, 'with reliance on severe splitting, expelling, and disowning' (p. 11). Brady movingly describes the abiding experiences of invisibility and insubstantiality that haunt the sense of being for anorexic teenagers. With equal compassion and insight, she provides compelling accounts of the manic defences that an adolescent may develop in the midst of a depressed and unresponsive family environment. This was the state of mind, body and being when Sara sought therapy for herself. She had become what Brady refers to as an 'unjoined person' (p. 8) for whom, 'feeling cut off from one's own or others' minds can leave chaotic emotions to be played out on the body' (p. 9). At the time Sara began therapy, she was severely anorexic. I struggled with my countertransferential fears that she could inadvertently destroy herself. I struggled to not get lost in efforts to get her to control her eating, but rather to help her establish more a vigorous relationship to her body and emotions.

Sara had approached me for therapy after two deeply troubled years in college, when her eating disordered behaviour was well established. Her mother did not want her to go into therapy (certainly not with me), but Sara sought me out as she remembered me from the TA for Teens class and my work with her brother, which she thought helped him. Our initial years of work were a combination of her participation in a TA therapy group and intensive neo-Reichian body-centred workshops, interspersed with individual sessions. I recall our using an image of hers being a 'picture window family', referring to the style of middle-class suburban housing that featured a large 'picture' window at the front of the house, opening into the living room, in which everything was on public display in a 'picture-perfect' fashion. Sara recalls our using the phrase 'postcard family', both of which present a picture-perfect family as viewed by others. By then in private practice, I was still a young, relatively inexperienced therapist and found the depth and persistence of Sara's obsessional concerns and eating patterns quite frightening. I managed to hold my countertransference in check and focused on trying to help Sara both recognize the severity of problems in her family while establishing a more positive attitude toward her body. The body-centred therapy involved regular touch which was intended to provide an experience of touch that was not punitive, but rather informative; it also allowed her expression of negative feelings that has been forbidden in her family. Her involvement in a long-term transactional analysis treatment group was extremely beneficial as a means of personal insight. In the group she felt less alone, she witnessed other people struggling with their own emotional issues, and she began to see the problems in her family with much more clarity.

As her therapy progressed and Sara worked desperately hard to establish life as an adult woman, more manic defences moved into the foreground. She studied, worked, walked, exercised non-stop, fighting off the depressive (and murderous) legacy of her family. I often found myself simultaneously alarmed and admiring of Sara's relentless activities, finding myself thinking that while she seemed half mad, I also found delight in her stubborn determination to make an independent life. My negative countertransference reactions shifted to hatred and contempt for her parents, her mother in particular. As I write now, I recall my associations at the time to Green's (1986) essay, 'The Dead Mother': '... that of an imago which has been constituted in the child's mind, following maternal depression, brutally transforming a living object, which was a source of vitality for the child, into a distant figure, toneless, practically inanimate ...' (p. 142). 'She [the dead mother] had been buried alive, but her tomb itself had disappeared. The hole that gaped in its place made solitude dreadful. As though the subject ran the risk of being sunk in it, body and possessions' (pp. 154–5).

I felt a deep, compelling identification with Sara as I, too, was dealing with the life-long impact of my mother's depressive collapse. My own analysis gave my compassion and understanding for what Sara was up against, and supervision provided the necessary distance to avoid collusion and an over-identification, which threatened to collapse the therapeutic space. For Sara, 'perfection' loomed again and again, working against her own self-understanding and compassion. Now, years later, as I read Brady's book (Brady, 2016), I've gained additional insights into Sara's dilemma at that time. Brady links the manic defences of adolescence and early adulthood to 'a central unconscious phantasy of a manic and self-destructive self in relation to an oblivious object' (p. 75). Sara's mother was in fact an 'oblivious' object, seemingly unable or unwilling to comprehend and take action with regard to severity of the life struggles her children faced. Sara was cast on her own to find a way to forge a life for herself.

An oblivious mother and an attentive therapist

B: When you look back over our work, what is your experience as what was really useful in our work, how things changed.

S: The first thing that came to my mind when I started looking back was 'chronicity'. You said over and over again, when I asked why I was having such a hard time, that through my whole childhood, adolescence and while we were working, the family process was the same. It was the chronicity – that's the word you kept using – of the damage, of how my mother was, of the lies and denial. That was all I ever knew. But you kept describing how this made my mind and my body so restricted and afraid to change. And then I thought it was the opposite kind of chronicity that you provided. You said things over and over again, as often as needed, with no blame, no shame. I always felt ashamed. My family had a history of mental illness, and my parents believed that mental illness was genetic. I believed that in every cell of my body. There was nothing that could be done about it. There was Larry. And I was to be their only hope. I had to be perfect. The vomiting had something to do with that. I had to get rid of the bad parts of me. I had to be whole, perfect.

There was a horror and disavowal within Sara's family of mental illness. Her brother was seen as schizophrenic, 'incurable', with all the disturbance projected into and onto faulty genetic material. Sara's reflections on the 'chronicity' that I offered her mirror Garfield's observations of the transformation of unbearable affect:

> As recovery from psychosis takes place, emotion combines more easily with the other two parts of the tripartite mind, cognition and the will. No longer must ones' thoughts [or emotions] be interpreted in a rigid fashion. Now, possibilities exist and there is less pressure to foreclose on alternatives. It is safe to come out of hiding; it is OK to share the boat with the therapist crewmate, especially within the therapeutic relationship.
>
> Garfield (2009, pp. 156–7)

S: Probably the primary technique we applied through the entire arc was for me to try to interrupt instant discharge activities at least long enough to try to identify feelings/thoughts, write them down. Initially I brought them all to our sessions to process, slowly/slowly sometimes I could figure out what childhood strictures I had violated or what current experience reminded me of some horror, and I could at least decrease the violence of the catharsis.

And then there was your warmth. You went way beyond the usual constraints of being a therapist. Your hugs. Your office was an adjunct to your house when I first started seeing you. Your office was like a home. I could see glimpses of a home, family, nothing like what I had known. Do you remember when your son was writing 'wolf' or 'the wolf' on slips of paper and leaving them everywhere? [My son renamed himself 'Scott the Wolf' for a year or so and left signs on his new name everywhere. We had insisted that the school allow him to sign his papers as 'Scott the Wolf'.] I remember finding these papers in the books and magazines in your waiting room, you explaining it to me. Charming!

As Sara and I looked back over her therapy, I was struck by her describing 'the primary technique' as being one of interrupting her 'instant discharge activities long enough to identify feelings/thoughts'. The quality and consistency of my attentiveness to her felt experience was central to our work. I did not address the dynamics of our relationship, though clearly my way of being with her was foundational, but rather kept my attention on her troubled relationship to her body and emotions. Although I did not know it at the time, I can see now that intuitively I was sustaining a primary focus of the vertical axis rather than horizontal (Lombardi, 2007; Lombardi and Pola, 2010; Goldberg, 2020).

Theoretical interlude: welcoming the sensate/somatic domains

Freud's early work was deeply rooted in his efforts to understand bodily experience, physical symptoms, sexuality and trauma. At the risk of seriously oversimplifying the complex evolution of Freud's thinking, I do wonder whether his distinction between 'actual' neuroses (which he identified as 'neurasthenia, anxiety neurosis, and hypochondria' (1917/1963, p. 390)) and psychoneuroses played a key role in his seeming to turn his attention away from the body and its myriad mysteries. He concluded, 'The problems of "actual" neuroses, whose symptoms are probably generated by direct toxic damage, offer psycho-analysis no points of attack. It can do little towards throwing light on them and must leave the task to biologico-medical research.' (p. 389)

Laplanche and Pontalis (1973) observed, 'From the therapeutic standpoint, the upshot of these views is that the actual neuroses cannot be treated psycho-analytically because their symptoms do not have a meaning that can be elucidated' (p. 10) but went on to note that 'the concept of actual neurosis is tending to disappear from present-day nosography' (p. 11). Whatever may be the reasons, over time, Freud came to privilege mind over body, language over action and affect, a perspective that has been the foundation of the theory and practice of American ego psychology and psychoanalysis. It has been left to others to bring psychoanalytic investigations to somatically based patterns of defence.

Reich (1949), in the development of character analysis, sought to reverse the Freudian order, arguing that verbal and cognitive processes are inevitably woven so deeply into the warp and woof of characterological and somatic defences as to all too often thwart classical analytic techniques. For Reich, consistent and subtle observations of bodily modes of expression and direct interventions at a body level were essential to the deep resolution of characterological defences. My early training in neo-Reichian models of psychotherapy has been invaluable to me. I learned to use my eyes and my hands, as well as my ears and my voice, in gathering information about my clients' ways of being – or not being – in relationship to their bodies. I learned how to make use of informed touch to access and accompany non-verbal domains (Cornell, 2015, 2016). I learned to welcome, rather than calm or avoid, deep states of affect. Garfield (2009), drawing upon Semrad's (Semrad and Van Buskirk, 1969) groundbreaking perspective on the role of affect in treating psychotic defences, observed:

> Semrad's second step, 'bearing affect' is a complex affair. It requires more than bringing the unbearable affect in

psychosis into the patient's body. ... Here the analyst is not only the co-pilot, but also, at times, serves as the patient's *own* missing eyes, ears, and hands. The therapist becomes, in some respects, a living part of the patient's experience.

Garfield (2009, p. ix, italics in original)

Although I did not have a deeply informed understanding of psychotic defences during the early years of my work with Sara, I did often experience my use of my body as a 'healthier' adjunct to Sara's, much as described by Garfield.

Within the models of psychotherapy based in Reich's work, the body was approached predominantly as a structure for defence – muscular and character armour. With some clients, this approach was highly effective, while with others it was severely disorganizing, sometimes I began to think, even damaging. I discovered the writings of Winnicott and Bollas, gradually coming to a different understanding of the means of relating to my clients' troubled, 'defended' bodies. Reading Winnicott and consulting with Bollas radically changed aspects of how I positioned myself as therapist in relation to my clients' patterns of bodily defences, changes which became evident in my work with Sara.

Winnicott (1950/1992) described 'reactions to impingement' in which the developing body learns to increasingly move *away from*, rather than *toward* the environment and others, so as to preserve some sense of self that could not be overtaken by the intrusive needs of others. Winnicott described this process as the creation of a false self – mirrored in Orbach's concept of false body and in Goldberg's later accounts of fabricated bodies. In the face of even more severe intrusive, violent, and/ or chaotic environments, a child 'then develops an extension of the shell rather than the core' (Winnicott, 1950/1992, p. 212). This was certainly true of Sara. Here I could find echoes of Reich's accounts of destructive family and social environments that necessitated the evolution of armour – a protective shell, but in Winnicott there was a more finely tuned sensitivity to the vulnerabilities that underlay the shell – a sensitivity that was often lacking in Reich's approach and in my original Reichian training. I needed to stop hammering on the shell, confronting defences, and find better means of access to the disowned, dissociated core of the self, as Winnicott (1964/1989) observed, "Am I beginning to convey my meaning that in practice there does exist a real and insuperable difficulty, the dissociation in the patient, as an organized defence, keeps separate the somatic dysfunction and the conflict in the psyche? Given time and favorable circumstances the patient will tend to recover from the dissociation" (p.106).

Bollas (1987, 1992) offered a radically different understanding of character. I have written elsewhere at length (Cornell, 2015, pp. 73–97) about the impact of Winnicott and Bollas on my ways of thinking about and working with characterological, i.e. unconscious, somatic defences and modes of experience.

Building a basement

S: Vomiting turned into DIRT. Shame became an inanimate object, dirt, that was everywhere. It provided a visceral relief. I was getting all the badness out. And I was getting praised for losing weight. It was a sequence, all connected. Eating disorders, exercise, OCD [Obsessive-Compulsive Disorder], dirt. Lurking underneath was this bodily soup that was always threatening to pull me under. Each iteration was some way to make it controllable. Each iteration was a little less harmful than the one before it. In my house growing up, I had no efficacy in anything, other than this. In these I thought I had some kind of control. I had to find control. Each was less dangerous. The dirt was outside.

Our work built a basement. You kept helping me see that my OCD, the anxieties there, were not real. You kept linking them to events, emotions, my past. You helped me see that there were triggers. You kept up a chronicity of correction to the chronicity of the damage. When I got too scared, you would call. I was not shamed for being in trouble.

As Sara and I talked together preparing for this paper, I could revisit the evolution of our therapeutic work in very much the sequence she described here – except that I had found her profound pre-occupation with **DIRT** to be almost unbearable. After her account of one incident of a frantic ridding of their house of 'dirt' – following a visit by her husband's family – I labelled her thinking and behaviour, bluntly, as psychotic. My terse and intense intervention both shocked and relieved her. It was the beginning of Sara being able to see that the physical manifestations of 'dirt' was actually a manifestation of feelings she couldn't tolerate.

I had by this time in the course of my work with Sara also discovered the work of Bucci (1997, 2001) and her articulation of the 'referential process' through which differing modes of psychic organization – verbal symbolic, non-verbal symbolic and subsymbolic – were gradually integrated into a more coherent whole of self-experience:

> It is necessary first to build connections within the nonverbal system between subsymbolic somatic activation and images of objects before meaningful verbal communication can occur. ... To the extent that physiological activation associated with strong emotion occurs without corresponding activation of cognitive contents in either initial or displaced form, thus without symbolic focus and regulation, the activation is likely to be prolonged and repetitive, and the ultimate effects on physiological systems to be more severe.
>
> Bucci (1997, p. 165)

Bucci's singular article crystalized intuitive understandings and changes I'd been struggling to make since first encountering Winnicott and Bollas. Her writing had a profound impact on my somatic work, resulting in a shift in how I worked with Sara and others. The Reichian-based models had a two-pronged focus: the confrontation of rigid muscular/characterological defences and an emphasis on emotional discharge. The referential process described by Bucci was much more intrapsychically focused with primary attention to the dissociative patterns that interrupted the flow and integration of experience among the three domains of psychic organization she described.

S: Something changed in your way of working. [Here is the influence that Winnicott, Bollas, and Bucci were having on my ways of working.] I had all these terrible feelings In the Radix [neo-Reichian] work the emphasis was on getting feeling OUT. That was a lot like what I was doing with the vomiting. Something changed. It was more about acceptance of trouble, acceptance of the defences. For me to learn to take in, rather than get it out. Radix was like the vomiting. There wasn't enough vomiting in the world to get rid of what was inside me. Then it was like you would say, 'Yes, it feels like dirt. It is not dirty. What are you feeling?' There was more about going inside myself, to say with myself, what I was feeling. You never shamed me.

You let me question you. You allowed my need to question you, to challenge you. [One of the members of Sara's therapy group made a serious suicide attempt, trying to kill himself in a devastating car wreck. I arranged for the group to continue meeting in the hospital so that he could be a part of the group while recovering.] When he was in the hospital, I began to hesitate about you, not trust if you knew what you were doing. I didn't want to say that, but I had to. You let me talk. You said that with my background [Dad and Larry's deaths] these were necessary questions. You were so honest. It was like you were telling me that I did have a brain, a good one. My feelings changed through questioning you. It was deeply affirming. I asked you if you knew what you were doing. You were so honest.

Sara's evolution of her sexual self

Sara's first date was her freshman year in college. During her high school years, given the violence she had witnessed from her brother and father, she was scared of boys. She described herself in high school as an 'ice princess'. 'I wanted to be admired but not touched. I had no feel of my sexuality.' Her high school years were rife with rejection and struggle, none of which seemed to be noticed by her mother. There was no discussion regarding sexuality. Sara was alone, and her body became the focus of her anxieties and efforts at self-control. Her first date was through the invitation of one young man on behalf of his friend who had been watching Sara around campus and wanted to take her to a formal dance. This young fellow also asked Sara if she would also kiss his friend. She accepted the dance but declined the kiss.

When Sara first began to live on her own, she lived with a man her age as roommates. He was an engineer and as described by Sara very methodical and goal-directed. He had a good job, a place to live, and so he needed a girlfriend (not Sara). He sent 21 postcards to women looking for someone to date through *Pittsburgh Magazine* (this was long before the internet) and succeeded. Sara followed suit with postcards of her own. The man she met was not to be in her life for more than a couple of dates. As we looked back, Sara said, 'I had a lot of first dates.' Her vomiting stopped while she lived with her roommate. During these years, her participation in the long-term TA group was crucial. There she found support, a place to talk about dating and sexuality, and the discovery that she was by no means alone in her insecurities and vulnerabilities in seeking a romantic and sexual life.

The first man she lived with as a sexual partner was, in Sara's words, 'A stable male presence, but quite parental – our anxieties didn't mesh.'

S: This was a move toward my first 'family'. But I felt I would never be fully accepted – if my own family didn't love me, no one would. Sex with him was nice – fun, enjoyable, rather lusty. He wanted me to do all the female roles, and this I resented. He liked my body, but that didn't change how I felt about my body. Something I understand now but didn't then is that I didn't have a measure of my body. I felt fat. I had to put on pants to see if they fit and get a sense of my size. I never used my body to attract men – make-up, etc. – that always made me uncomfortable – it was scary. It's heartbreaking, how I had to control my emotions, push away what was wrong with me. I was able to make him happy rather than enjoying my own body. My body was closed to me. His rigidity set off my OCD. My vomiting had stopped, I put on weight, and that's when the 'dirt' started.

'Dirt' became a certain focus of our work for several years. Headway was slow. Sara experimented with cognitive-behavioural treatments for her OCD to complement what we were doing. I was open to anything that might give her help, but she found little relief or change in these approaches. Her trust was with me, and it was my job to manage my own anxieties and continue to focus on her gaining more tolerance and understanding of the raw emotions that her constant cleaning sought to manage and purge.

I silently admired Sara's determination to have a sexual life, which at the time seemed to me to defy all the odds for someone with her adolescence and such a troubled relationship to her body. I kept my hope and admiration for her efforts to myself, so as to preserve her sexual explorations as her own, not an adaptation to please me. I was dismayed at the intensification of her OCD and overwhelming preoccupation with dirt and cleaning. Throughout our work I sought to keep my (and sometimes her own) focus on her internal relationship to herself, her emotions and her body, to be able to grasp how her OCD cut her off from what was actually disturbing her, silencing the voice of disturbance and meaning.

Sara was briefly involved with a man to whom she was 'wildly attracted' and with whom she felt a freedom to experiment. Their sexual relationship was great, and sex was their primary bond. She became pregnant but miscarried, which was profoundly painful for her. 'He didn't have the emotional maturity to help me, so we said goodbye.' Her next relationship was to the man, also met through a magazine advert, who was to become her husband, now for over 20 years.

> S: He was a gentleman. He didn't push for sex, saying he wanted to savour getting to know me. He said we had both needed 'practice people' beforehand, so that we could really appreciate each other. He had watched the pain his father had caused his mother and sisters, and he had hurt some of the women he'd been with. He had a strong sexual drive, so he hadn't always been so kind with other women. He was kind and respectful with me. His kindness truly benefited me.

After about ten years in this relationship, Sara decided to return to school and pursue a programme to become a Physician's Assistant. During the programme she became 'an angry, ornery mess'; she hated the programme, the rigidity and authoritarian attitudes of the faculty throwing her back into a world where it felt like her father was lurking around every corner. 'My husband had the emotional maturity to stay with me through it all.' Again, she persisted, and these were the turbulent emotional waters into which the new man in her life was thrown. Sara had come to minimize any direct contact with her own family, in an effort to ward off their intrusiveness. Her husband-to-be, however, maintained contact with his family (who lived several hours away) and they welcomed Sara into their lives. This was not easy for her. Being with his family evoked intense anxiety, the feelings of being intruded upon, with the inevitable escalation of her war against 'dirt'. He asked if he could attend some of her sessions. This was not to be some form of couples counselling, but a request on his part to gain a better understanding of therapy and what she was struggling with. He rarely said a word, simply sat quietly, listening, often holding her hand, watching how I listened and spoke to Sara. It was a rather unique, and definitely productive, sort of therapeutic encounter.

> S: Of all the men I've been with, he says over and over again how much he likes my body. The things we talked about in this room about my body began to feel real in my head, but I couldn't hold it in my body. The impact of his body, his kindness, and his sexual interest in me – the things you and I built were good but with my husband it has become real in my body. He has always focused on my pleasure, and my body does respond. He is the most thoughtful, loving partner I have had. From the start there was much more depth to our connections: sharing observations, appreciations, challenges so the physical relationship started with more nuance. Still, I wish I could bring my body more fully to him. It has to do with the splitting I had to do to survive. It's still here. I often watch the world.

Looking back

It was fascinating to hear Sara, as we sat in my office looking back over the years of our work together, speak of the changes she noticed in my ways of working. These changes were never addressed directly as I worked with Sara and others (something that I very likely would do now), and yet they registered with her in significant ways. There was a quiet, but palpable intimacy between us as we shared our memories and reflections.

Sara and I worked together on and off for over 30 years. Each time she made a major step forward into her own life, one she had chosen and typically worked incredibly hard to achieve, there would be a return of anxiety and the impulse to return to obsessional ways of coping. It was as though, each time, her mind and reflective capacities would disappear, and her sensate/motoric body would take over. Together, over the years, Sara and I learned to be less alarmed by the return of these life-long coping mechanisms, which gradually lost most of their obsessional, anxiety-drenched grip on her ways of being. We came to see them as distress signals warning of the imagined (and remembered) risks of her taking another step toward making her life her own – a psychological, unconscious transgression of her family's strictures. We were able to hold the dynamic tension between the defensive *and* the communicative functions of her relationship to food, her OCD, dread of dirt and compelling need to be 'perfect'. She has been able to transform her preoccupations with her own body into a skilled and successful medical career, working as a compassionate physician's assistant specializing in nutrition. She has sustained a loving, physically intimate relationship for more than two decades, declaring herself the luckiest women in the world to be with the man she loves. She still thinks about writing.

CHAPTER 9

Responding to trauma-based communication in psychotherapy

Mark Linington

Introduction

> If our supposition is correct, a comparison between the psychology of primitive peoples, as it is taught by social anthropology, and the psychology of neurotics, as it has been revealed by psycho-analysis, will be bound to show numerous points of agreement and will throw new light upon familiar subjects.
>
> Freud (1912–1913, p. 1)

> The split between ego and id, or between rationalisation and desire, is distinctly historical. It is the domination of nature carried inward, to 'human nature' itself, now defined as an ego that hates its 'animal' id. The products of this inner fission react upon another to produce Freud's superego, and bad conscience. And the bad conscience of the west reacts upon its dominated dark peoples to generate white racism. Since, however, these processes are set going all at the same time, it is also the case that white racism generates the characteristic form of the western imperial psyche. That is why the id is black, and why the superego hates the thing it is driven to save.
>
> Kovel (1988, p. cviii)

It is now perhaps impossible to use the word and concept 'primitive' in any context without an awareness of its historically racist and colonial use, and the horrifying actions which it has supported. Certainly, the use of the word in the field of anthropology has been criticized (Boas, 1911), as it has also been in regard to art (Antliff and Leighten, 2003). The problem is not solved by the idealization of 'the primitive' which one finds in concepts such as primitivism in art and in anarcho-primitivist political theory. But within psychoanalysis, the use of the word to this day persists (e.g. Eekhof, 2019; Van Buren and Alhanti, 2010), as though it is not only unproblematic, but also elucidating. We could think that the word primitive in psychoanalytic thinking is merely a synonym for 'early' – describing the ways in which the infant relates to others, but it is more than that. It is also a term that relates to a developmental trajectory, in which we move up a hierarchy of increased sophistication from a state of immaturity to maturity, from the primitive to the civilized. Within psychoanalysis, the 'primitive' is characterized by a concern with primitive emotional states (murderous rage, hate and terror) and primitive ways of being and communicating in relationships (projection, omnipotence, idealization, projective identification), with the espoused aim of psychoanalysis being to acculturate through thinking such primitive processes.

We might be ashamed if we thought we were partaking as psychotherapists in an enterprise underlaid by such a dehumanizing and white Eurocentric paradigm. We might wish to distance ourselves from this aspect of psychoanalysis by doubting the presence of such unconscious racism tangled up in our theoretical foundations. However, there can be less doubt that the word 'primitive', although apparently empirically descriptive, is used pejoratively in relationships. When I was told on my own psychotherapy training that I was expressing myself primitively, it was not, I think, a positive acknowledgement. I was being uncivilized, with a history of meaning packed up tight in the word *primitive* itself.

But in saying this, I have no wish to throw out the psychoanalytic baby with the racist bathwater. Attention to murderous rage and hate, and to implicit relational and embodied communications through processes such as projection, and so on, is a vital part of psychotherapy. Attention is essential particularly to the non-verbal and bodily ways feelings, most often 'unfelt feelings' (Orbach, personal communication), and unconscious relational patterns, the 'unthought known' (Bollas, 1987), are present in current adult relationships, if we are to help people in a profound and sustainable way. Furthermore, there are two notions that may not be acknowledged in this crypto-colonial thinking:

1. That the content and forms of such communications are not genetic, but rather epigenetic. In other words, our persistent murderous rage is not an innate death instinct (Freud, 1920), but rather a response to the experienced reality of the frightening aspects of our earliest attachments. Murderous rage, hate and terror and the projective characteristics of the form of our communication are a response to trauma in attachment relationships.
2. That the helpful psychotherapeutic task is not the eradication or civilizing of these so-called primitive communications through the imperious wisdom of our interpretations and insight, but the bringing of these aspects of ourselves into a securer, more felt and conscious relationship with the other longer-lived body-based selves, through a relational experience with an empathic caregiver.

Below I give two clinical examples, in which I will refer to 'primitive' bodily communications as trauma-based communication or 'unfelt feelings'. These clinical examples will illustrate something of this area of work with trauma-based early communication, including considerations of the links between such emotional communication and interpersonal traumatic experience, the significance of the impact of such communications on the psychotherapist, and some discussion about how transformation begins to happen.

Sue: Communicating the horror of trauma[1]

> Horror is the uncanny emotion that all of you have known at least once, probably in your sleep. Horror is a simply paralyzing combination of what I like to call revulsion – a feeling of almost total desire to be elsewhere and away from all this sort of thing – coupled again with a great desire to vomit, and perhaps a tendency to have diarrhoea and one thing and another; and at the same time there is literally a sort of paralysis of everything, so that nothing really goes on except this awful and – if it can possibly be avoided – never-to-be-repeated-experience.
>
> Sullivan (1953, p. 316)

When a referral arrives where I work, and we discuss it as colleagues, I often find myself powerfully drawn to working with people who have experienced the most horrible trauma. In this therapeutically heroic zeal to care (Searles, 1979), there is a lot of my own self material. This is present together with a picking up of the transferential communications that seem to come with most referrals. From my side, there is at least sometimes, a perhaps masculine desire to show off my special power, mixed both with an identification with the hurt person and the activation of my natural caregiving instincts as a keystone system (McCluskey and O'Toole, 2020). So, this time, it stood out like a sore thumb, when, from the first I heard of Sue, I felt horror and revulsion and wanted to stay well away from any work with her.

Sue was an Afro-Caribbean woman in her fifties, from London, with Down's syndrome. She had a diagnosis of severe learning disability and another of bipolar affective disorder. Although she was not believed to have epilepsy, she was having some sort of seizures. These were being medically investigated at the time she was referred. She used limited language but was described as understanding things well. In the tone of this description there was the suggestion that perhaps she was withholding something from her relating: as though her adoption of a secondary handicap (Sinason, 1992) was an attack on the world. She was described in the referral as having been depressed for the last six months. Her depression had been accompanied by what were called 'significant behavioural problems'. These included: screaming and shouting, throwing objects, repeated regurgitation, spitting and faecal smearing. It was as though everything horrible was coming out of her. Often, in my experience, when people with learning disabilities express themselves in such ways, it is understood still, as the lack of social restraint, the unleashing of the primitive instincts onto the world, with no developed ego to hold back the marauding id. Such is the drive theory model that many people with learning disabilities still have to endure. The people who worked with Sue were described as not liking her, finding her very difficult to be with and she was constantly attacking them. She had been banned from the day centre where she had been going for a number of years, because the staff there could not cope with her aggressive behaviour.

Sue was abandoned by her parents at the very beginning of her life. It is not known whether this was after she was identified as having Down's syndrome or not. But many parents have reported the difficulty of receiving the news that their child has a disability (Korff-Sausse, 1999). In the late 1950s, as a baby, Sue was put into an asylum for the mentally handicapped, with around a thousand other people, where she stayed for more than thirty years. In the early 1990s, when she came out, she was in her thirties. She was moved into a staffed community home, as part of the institution closure programme. From the beginning, most staff and other residents did not like her much and she had a series of different behavioural interventions to try and stop her aggressive outbursts. Staff complained that they could not be consistent with her in carrying out these interventions, because she liked some of them more than others. Staff did talk about Sue's sense of humour. This humour showed itself in the form of mimicking other residents, which often upset the residents, but sometimes amused the staff. Sue was said to become aggressive when she did not have attention from a member of staff. Her aggression could sometimes take the form of self-harm (banging her head and tearing at her skin), as well as smashing things and hitting people. While she was in this home she was sexually abused by a male member of staff, who left the home as a result. It was about this time that she was diagnosed with bipolar disorder and given medication. A couple of years later, her violence towards others and property had reached the point where she was sectioned and put into hospital. She stayed in this hospital for about a year for assessment and treatment and then came out into a different community home.

Much of the detail of Sue's history has been lost. This lack of history in itself generates a vicious lack of subjectivity. As psychotherapists, with an understanding of attachment theory, we know the difficulties it can cause for a person, if they do not have their own formulated narrative available to them. This lack of a narrative may influence others, including staff, to treat a person more as an object. A person is much more likely to be a subject for others where they possess their own narrative. For Sue, the availability of this narrative is further hampered – but not made impossible – both by her lack of verbal language and her living with unresolved multiple traumas.

The first time I met Sue was the second appointment I had offered. The staff, who worked with her in her residential home, had told me that they had forgotten about the first appointment. As she shuffled out of the lift, with a staff member on either side of her, she looked desolate and squalid, quite worn out. Her clothes – T-shirt and tracksuit bottoms

– seemed to have been selected for their muddy-coloured formlessness. There seemed no person there to meet. She was entirely not the raging, horrifyingly uncontained primitive-monster, I had feared might come tearing out at me. Her dark greasy hair stuck to her head. I looked, and could not tell whether she had Down's syndrome or not: I felt so unsure that I thought I might have been mistaken in my memory, about what I had understood of her disability. She somehow seemed too thin, sunken and indistinct to have something as definite as Down's syndrome. She was stooped over, like she was carrying some load and walked as though her feet were chained together. She frowned at me, half-hidden, from under her brows, all the time silent. All in all, she gave the impression of having been a prisoner for a long time. I suggested to Sue that we might go to the psychotherapy room, which was down the end of a long corridor. She immediately moved to come with me. Then as the two staff moved to follow her, I noticed her hesitate – as though she was unsure as to whom she belonged. As we moved off down the corridor we came to a locked door, which I needed to unlock. As I did this, Sue groaned and began to pull down her trousers. The staff moved quickly to stop her. I said to Sue that I thought it must be a bit frightening coming to this strange place, to see me, whom she did not know. I said perhaps we could see how she felt when we got to the room. I could see the staff smiling at each other in a sort of collusive way and felt embarrassed at having spoken to Sue as though she was an understanding person.

When we got to the room for this first session, the staff directed Sue to sit down in one of the chairs. The staff went to wait in another room nearby. Sue stood up and started making a wailing sound, like distressed sobbing; but with no tears. She sat down and then stood up again and began to take down her trousers. I said that I thought she was very upset and she wanted to let me know something important. She sat back down and sat turned away from me. She was silent and still for a while. Intermittently, she would part stand up, pull her trousers down a little and half put her hand down the back of her trousers onto her bottom. I said that I thought it was difficult being here with me. I said that she wanted to let me know about something. I said perhaps touching your bottom gives you a feeling. I had a horrible fearful image that kept coming to me, when she did this: that she might bring out her hand holding not just a fistful of shit, but a horrible handful of gory organs. I said this is frightening; I am thinking about what you are doing and how you feel. I said I am thinking about what people have done to you. She turned to look at me, full face, and screamed and spat. A glob of pale brown spittle went on to her front. I thought how small and pathetic it looked compared to the feeling she had communicated. She looked down at it for some moments. I looked at it and I felt disgusted. This gloop looked like an unsavoury sort of baby food. I said, I think you are spitting out something horrible.

She looked around the room, at the different things in it, particularly the dolls (I had four soft dolls dressed in a variety of clothes. A feature of these dolls is that underneath their clothes their genitals are represented). I said something to recognize her doing this. She looked at me and spat again – this time the spit reaching me, landing on my knee. I said that I thought she must be angry. She looked at me very directly and then seemed to relax a bit. She sat back in the chair. There was a long period of silence. I sat and looked at the spit on my leg and wondered what to do about it; I imagined Sue's stomach acid corroding a hole through my clothes. I regretted that I had worn my good suit to this session; but I decided to leave it there for now. After a while of sitting calmly, I offered a pad of paper to Sue and a few crayons and pencils. She looked at them and moved the crayons and pencils away and said, 'No'. She looked at the pad of paper, then vomited onto it a mouthful of the same brown regurgitation. I felt a rush of revulsion and panic. I could feel my mind and my body seizing up with a creeping paralysis. I was aware of standing back from myself in a sort of dissociative way. I wanted to shake myself and told myself to pull myself together. A thought came to mind, of how since I had become a parent I had been able to catch the vomit of my children. Sue sat looking away. I said something else has come out of her. She said, 'Look,' and put her finger into the sick. I noticed how neatly the splash of puke fitted onto the paper. She picked up the pad of paper and tried to turn it into my lap. I held the pad to keep it off me and we sat like this, in a sort of motionless combat, looking at each other face to face. I said I think you feel terrible. Sue looked away from me and vomited several times onto the floor. Some fell on her. She sat and looked for a while at the vomit around her. Then, she turned and looked at me and said, 'Cloth'.

I will stop here, before I go and get the cloth. This is an option in a chapter that is of course not available in the same way when we are with someone in psychotherapy. Even in the writing about this session for you, I have found it a tough test of my endurance. I would like to have come out of this session, on and off, throughout it. The room smelt terrible. There was sick all around. At any moment, I feared Sue might start slinging shit. I had moments where I wanted to shout, 'How could you do that!' and 'Get out of here!'

Despite this awful beginning, I did begin weekly psychotherapy with Sue. I first carried out four assessment sessions with Sue – which were, in one way, my attempt to try and understand and think seriously about whether psychotherapy was going to be of any help to her. In another way, these assessment sessions were also my delaying of a beginning with her. I wanted to hold her at a distance. But it did give me some hope that people said that Sue had been calmer since beginning her psychotherapy and was regurgitating, vomiting and stripping less. However, this was not likely to be a fairy-tale psychotherapy where I could chop through the forest to wake a sleeping beauty or transform the primitive beast with my enduring love. With its likelihood of eternally returning despair, this felt more like a job for Sisyphus. So, it was still with some trepidation that I began the psychotherapy – with the support of my supervisor and my surrounding colleagues. The purpose of the psychotherapy was, I think, to empathically recognize and understand Sue as a subject and to communicate my subjective understanding of her to her. Another way to say this is that we might move from an object to object relating (in which the objects enact much cruel persecution) to an intersubjective relating. When this intersubjective understanding and communication failed and relating again became trauma-based ('primitive'), I hoped that we would find enough security, vitality and newness (Shane, Shane and Gales, 1997) between us to sustain us in our relationship. I thought our first session had augured well for such surviving.

At the beginning, Sue arrived for our sessions looking very depressed. Sometimes she seemed not to recognize me when we met. I often felt entirely hopeless at this point – thinking I was utterly insignificant to her: that I held no place in her mind and had been forgotten. Feeling and understanding my despair seemed one route to understanding Sue. I thought of her experience of being forgotten. Every time in the session, there seemed sufficient connection between us to keep us both going. I became aware of how much I needed to be fed and sustained by the psychotherapy: that I needed a certain amount of lively connection to keep me going; lest the despair overtake me.

For the first few months of psychotherapy Sue would start the sessions, as soon as we got into the room, in an angry way: standing up and walking round the room shouting and screaming – but rarely saying any words except 'No' and 'Get out'; turning over tables and chairs and throwing the things across the room – like dolls, and the clock. I was not sure that she wanted to be there. I wondered whether the experience of psychotherapy with me, might feel to her threateningly like the sexual abuse she had had to endure with the male member of staff. I noticed that she did not throw anything directly at me. It seemed as though she wanted to say something about damage: to have it there, but that she was showing some concern in the way she was damaging. She never broke or tore anything, even in the most trauma-based moments. She never caused me any damage – beyond that small bit of spit on my nice suit. But I also knew I had strong feelings, a lot of the time, of wanting to be rid of her. So I tried to gently keep the limits of what damage could be caused, while at the same time recognizing the feelings she was communicating. During the middle of these sessions, Sue would most often calm and sit in the chair, or lie on the couch and look at me. She would sometimes look at me and scream; sometimes she fell asleep. I noticed she always woke before the end of the session and so took it as both an active and relieving (McCluskey, 2005) form of relating.

There was, perhaps inevitably, an issue about Sue missing me and me abandoning her. Often, as we neared the end of a session Sue would become angry again and would start throwing things and screaming. I noticed that despite the apparent limitations in the language that she spoke that she often seemed to listen to what I communicated and responded to it. So when I said that I thought she was finding it difficult saying goodbye, at the end of each session – with me having in mind her history of abandonment – she calmed. When we came to the lift to say goodbye, for the first time she held out her hand towards me, which I took and held for a few moments, as we said goodbye.

As we went on, Sue started to lie on the floor more in sessions. Sometimes she would lie on the couch. She would on occasions pull my chair over, so that it was nearer to the couch. Sometimes she would come and lie on the floor close to me. She would often assume what seemed like submissive sexual positions with her legs, or bottom, in the air, or on all fours. With her bottom aimed towards me, she would scream and wail. I felt like she was offering herself to me sexually and felt sick. I felt like an abuser and wanted it to stop. It was at this time, that she took one of the female anatomically detailed dolls, lifted up the skirt and retched over it – but no vomit came out. I said to her that I thought horrible things had been done to her body, by another person. I said these things made both of us feel sick; but it was important for me to know about these things that had been done to her. She wrapped herself in the rug and went to sleep on the floor.

In time it was confirmed that Sue had dementia. I felt outraged. Given the life that Sue had led and the experiences that had been dealt to her; given what had been so far difficult to build together in the psychotherapy, to have another enduring terrible experience felt designed as a crushing cruelty. That, further, I would not be able to necessarily know from Sue how this dementia was experienced by her and that she might not be able to know what was happening to her, I think added to the pain of the situation.

Sue was moved to a nursing home specializing in dementia. The staff started to bring Sue to her sessions in a wheelchair. She was usually asleep when she arrived, or lolling to the side, like she was semi-conscious. I found the feelings of despair and inadequacy that I often felt at the beginning of the sessions became intensified. But as soon as the staff left the room Sue would begin to stir and struggle to get out of the wheelchair. She would sometimes scream as she did this. She would get onto the floor, or onto the couch, sometimes wrap herself in the rug and close her eyes, seeming to sleep, often for most of the session. One time towards the end of our time together, she lay on the couch curled in a foetal position and cried and for the first time, I saw, she was crying tears.

On the day I returned to work from the summer break, Sue died. She was meant to come to her first session back that day. She died following a seizure brought on by her dementia. I was not entirely surprised by the timing of Sue's death. I had felt it in the air, as a possibility, as we had come to the break, knowing how difficult these separations were for her. I could not attend her funeral, which I found difficult and sad. I felt that I had betrayed her and been very cruel in my abandonment and these were – perhaps are – difficult feelings to be left with. I hoped that Sue had experienced at least an understanding soothing connection in the last months of her life, but this was not something I could know and this was a particularly difficult aspect of the work with her. Certainly she had become less primitively monstrous, not just for me, but in her relating with others and seemingly in her sense of self. But in losing her monstrousness, perhaps there was also lost her sense of strength in the world and this was painful. In some ways I felt culpable for her death and angry that she could have abandoned me. This work with Sue was highly significant for me, because in it she did become a person, not just a monster of behaviours, 'on whose nature, nurture could never stick' (Shakespeare 1623/1923 IV. i. 188–9). In becoming a subject in my mind, she became more a subject to herself. I think this was a probably a very difficult process for her: becoming more a person (with the mourning pain that came with that), at the same time as her dementia was probably taking away this sense of self and relationship. But despite this difficulty I think this psychotherapeutic relationship was of significant value.

There seem to be a number of features that emerge in working with someone who is communicating early experiences of abusive attachment trauma including:
1. The communication was made by the body in an enactive and relational way (Orbach, 2009).
2. There was a lack of verbal language. Although Sue reportedly had more verbal language than she used in the psychotherapy with me, it seemed the violent destructive physical communication she needed to represent her interpersonal abusive experiences had come to dominate her and her way of relating to others.
3. That the attempts to mirror (Winnicott, 1971) and then understand what is being communicated through the early body processes (vomiting, spitting, body movements, etc.) seemed to be relieving.

Primitive: unfelt feelings

in me that were without when the panting stops scraps of an ancient voice in me not mine
Beckett (1964, p. 7)

'Primitive' is one identity of many, for a person with a dissociative identity disorder (DID), mostly known as Vicky. Vicky reported, as did those who had worked with her previously, that she had several other adult and childlike identities often active in different ways in the external world. She said that she did not know all of these identities, but knew of them, often from things they did when she was in an unconscious dissociated state but became aware of later. Vicky was a small, thin, working-class woman in her sixties, who had spent much of her childhood in care, being moved from placement to placement, when relationships broke down, often after experiences of abuse at home. These were sometimes not known at the time, and when she had reported them, they were disbelieved and dismissed. Vicky frequently described how the hurt of not being believed and having her reality dismissed was as damaging as the abusive experiences themselves.

In addition, she had experienced prolonged ritualized sexual abuse in more than one institution. She described organized groups of men and women, who had carried out pseudo-religious ceremonies that incorporated the sexual abuse of several children. She had shown great determination in obtaining an education for herself and had later gone on to have a successful civil service career.

On first meeting Vicky for an assessment, she reported a continuous shouting and screaming inside herself coming from another identity called 'Primitive'. She said she had been hearing their voice throughout her life. She described it as an ancient and ungendered voice she had known since early childhood that was, she repeatedly assured me, definitely not hers. In this first meeting Vicky said she was scared to let Primitive talk with me because she was not sure what would happen. She thought it could be very dangerous, and she felt deeply ashamed to admit that she was possessed by what she thought of as a furious and out of control part of herself, that was not herself. She said that Primitive regularly harmed her body in horrible ways, but she was too frightened to describe these in any detail.

It seems to be a not infrequent phenomenon for people who are in the early stages of getting help with their dissociative identity disorder to have very difficult struggles with an identity that is a more severely punishing version of the anti-libidinal ego/internal saboteur (Fairbairn, 1952). Such identities seem to 'hold' traumatic memories and are often younger seeming and tempestuous in the way they relate. Sometimes the existence of such an identity is not consciously known by the person's main identity, called 'the host' or Apparently Normal Person (ANP) (van der Hart, Nijenhuis and Steele, 2006). The feelings (and the memories associated with these feelings) that are experienced and expressed by this internal saboteur are often not felt or known by other identities.

Vicky was referred to the psychotherapy clinic by her psychiatrist, because she was struggling with a number of dissociative identity disorder symptoms. These included: losing time, finding serious injuries to her body, a sense of her body not being entirely hers, and the world about her not feeling real. She would find herself in places with no memory of how she had got there and hear a screaming voice inside her head. As stated, she knew that she had other identities from evidence she had found but had no real sense of what these identities were like or what they did. She referred to these identities as 'heteronyms', although she did not know where she had learned this unusual word. 'Heteronyms', is a term coined by Fernando Pessoa (Pessoa, 1991), a Portuguese writer from the early twentieth century, to describe his many different identities. It is not clear where Vicky had learned this word. It was possible it might have been a coincidental coining. However, from later conversations, it seemed that one or more of her identities may have been researching the nature of DID. She often found childlike drawings lying around her flat and sometimes she had a sense of having travelled somewhere (and could verify this on her car mileage). She told me what she knew in a general way about her history of serious sexual abuse, frequently carried out by people who were attachment figures in her life. She said this abuse had begun in her early teenage years when she was living in care, although we were later to discover that she had had much earlier abusive experiences in her birth family and in organized groups. Vicky had no memory of these earlier experiences, and it was to become clear that the memories of abuse that she did have were missing many of the most horrific details.

In addition, she described struggling with a number of functional issues, including falling into a sort of freeze state, meaning she could often not go out, or complete the most basic tasks at home, including eating and drinking, going to the toilet and sleeping. She said these states could last for long periods. She reported that there was regular harm, through cutting, to her body. She said it she knew was Primitive who stopped her doing these activities and who carved words on her body.

When Vicky began twice-a-week psychotherapy with me, it was predominantly Vicky who would be present in the sessions. Occasionally a distressed and scared child identity would be present, who would cry and rock and need soothing. Mostly these sessions were used by Vicky to describe ongoing battles inside with Primitive, who stopping her doing things by bringing on a frozen state and emerging at times to harm her body.

For the first three months of their psychotherapy, Primitive did not appear in the psychotherapy, although Vicky would often tell me about hearing them shouting inside, often commenting in negative ways about Vicky and how weak and useless she was, about how they wanted to kill her and furiously criticizing me and the therapy. Vicky reported that sometimes she would find that words had been etched with a sharp implement into different places on her body: words like 'whore', 'hate', 'rage' and 'die'. On occasions Primitive had tried to kill her by taking her to a bridge and threatening to jump off. Somehow at moments before this was enacted, Vicky or another identity had emerged and been able to stop the attempt. On several occasions the police had had to be involved.

Twice in the first three months Primitive came out in the psychotherapy sessions. They emerged screaming that they hated Vicky and me and that they were going to kill Vicky. They would glare fiercely, though never at me face to face, and sometimes make slow steps forward, tangentially approaching nearer to me, with their fists clenched, as though they were going to attack. As they approached in this indirect manner, I noticed how – not unlike the work with Sue – saying something recognizing, such as, 'I can see how you are full of horrible feelings; I think you are trying to get rid of them' would seem to halt them. They would hit the body, saying, 'This is not my body, it is Vicky's body,' banging the head, genitals and chest shouting, 'I hate it, I hate it!' then start punching the walls and throwing furniture and other things in the room. They threw the four soft dolls around the room, having looked and seen their genitals, and stamped on them repeatedly. The body's face at this time was contorted with feeling of hate. I am saying 'the body' here because Primitive did not experience the body as their own. They saw themselves as not having a body. This is a not uncommon phenomenon for some identities of a person with DID. It seems likely that it is a way of managing the horrific experiences of severe repeated childhood sexual abuse. How to bring them into a relationship with the body as *their* body and a *shared* body, shared between identities, is an important part of the work. For example, Primitive went into a flashback of an abusive experience when I first asked them to look at the body and see if they could connect with it in some way. I was too precipitate in trying to work in this way – hoping to find some means to use a connection with their body to help them regulate the intensity of their feelings. Very frightening flashbacks threatened to overwhelm them. However, fortunately, I managed to repair this with them, by acknowledging my mistake, and us understanding more together about why such a connection felt so painful and overwhelming. The development of such a connection came about much later in the work.

I could feel a fear rising strongly into me at these times where Primitive was raging. Predominantly, I experienced this feeling of fear in my body: sweating, increased heart rate, nausea and quickened shallow breathing. I sometimes felt very small, sometimes I would feel murderously destructive.

Six months into the therapy with Vicky, Primitive wrote to me by email for the first time. The email was a torrent of invective, full of rage and hate, saying they wanted to kill Vicky because of the things she had done in the past and that they wanted to kill me because the therapy I was doing with Vicky was giving her feelings, and they were starting to feel these more intensely too. They hated me for making them feel. They described these feelings as a 'big mass'. I responded that I thought they had been courageous to talk with me and that it must be an awful experience to be full of so much horrible feeling. They said that they hated feeling feelings. I wondered whether they would like to write to me more often, at a regular time, and wondered if this might be easier initially than coming to see me in the therapy room. Somewhat surprisingly, they said they would like to do this. We began a process of writing to each other once a week for a set time period (50 minutes).

Primitive communicated with me once a week by email for a further eighteen months. For a time their emails were full of fury, expressing their desire to be rid of all of these hateful and hated feelings. I concentrated in the first place on recognizing these feelings, mirroring them back verbally to them without any seeking to transform or to defend against them (Winnicott, 1971). My being able to engage in this way took significant support from others.

Primitive at this time reported to me that they did not find it easy to look at mirrors, as what they saw was someone who was not them and a body they did not recognize. As time went on, this relational mirroring process in itself became regulating, and often began to settle the rage that Primitive was feeling; although this was often unsustainable beyond the contact that we had together in the email. As time went on, with much repeated mirroring back of the feelings, Primitive began to express more interest in other feelings. They began to feel other feelings like sadness and eventually, after several months, to notice that they could feel joy. It is notable that as these interpersonal feeling developments began to take place, there was a parallel development in the telling of the story of multiple abusive traumas and a gradual coming to be able to accept the body as theirs as well as Vicky's.

The development by Primitive of being able to feel feelings, not just feelings of hate and murderous rage, but sadness, compassion and joy, seemed very significant. They developed an interest in understanding emotions, they became hungry for representing their emotional experience and started to explore creative ways of doing this (in drawings and poetry for example). The development of this capacity to feel their feelings rather than to disavow them, or to feel frighteningly overwhelmed by them, was significant, and I noticed that it was at this time that I began to enjoy the interactions with Primitive, despite the horrifying material. My feelings seemed to expand in tandem with theirs.

Around this time Primitive began to wonder about coming again to see me in person. They were particularly concerned to see my face so they could see how I was feeling when I was relating with them. We planned – together with Vicky – how Primitive might once again return to the in-person psychotherapy sessions.

The fissured relationship between Vicky and Primitive changed radically over the course of the psychotherapy, as they were able to meet each other and share more of their experiences. With help, they slowly got to understand each other better, initially almost entirely as separate people in a couple relationship. There was a change in the quality of conversation between them, characterized especially by increased empathy expressed towards each other. There is not space here to describe the details of this piece of ongoing couple work, which became in turn, a sort of group psychotherapy with other identities. It also seemed significant that Vicky began for the first time to develop in her ability to feel feelings. The relationship between them became increasingly collaborative and communication was no longer dominated by enacted screaming rage and fear. Primitive stopped harming the body. There was some sharing of the memories of the trauma (although it is likely that Vicky never knew the full details of traumas which Primitive was able to describe).

Discussion

There are a number of common features between the traumatized 'uncivilized' communication of Sue and Primitive. Both of them had undoubtedly experienced severe early and ongoing abusive trauma involving caregivers. In addition to these experiences of violence against their bodies, they had both had long experiences of neglect and the lack of another who would receive and return this communication of disorganized trauma-based feeling. As Winnicott (1971, p. 113) says, 'A baby so treated will grow up puzzled by mirrors and what the mirror has to offer'. The receiving of these feelings and their mirroring back in the most basic way, without any action to transform or civilize it, confirmed something about an aspect of their emotional reality and began the process of allowing the feelings to be felt. It is notable that in the work with both Sue and Primitive, it was initially unbearable for them to look directly into my face, this could only be done askance or avoided entirely; as though I was not going to mirror something back that would confirm their sense of self: 'getting back what they are giving' (Winnicott, 1971, p. 112).

A further key part of this transformational process, with Sue and Primitive, seems to have been the ability of the psychotherapist to receive and feel the feelings (of horror, rage and hate) that are as yet unfelt, as anything other than a 'big mass', by the person themself. During this time of intense caregiving, and a powerful activation of the most vulnerable aspects of my own internal environment, I had to work to develop and maintain my ability to seek care from others and share my experience of the work with supportive peers (McCluskey, 2005 and McCluskey and O'Toole, 2020). Without this network of intimate support, I would not have been able to sustain my secure-enough engagement in the work with Sue and Primitive.

Notes

1. An earlier version of this section previously appeared as part of a paper, in *Attachment: New Directions in Relational Psychoanalysis and Psychotherapy*, Linington (2009).

References

Foreword

Beebe, B. and Lachmann, F. (2002). *Infant Research and Adult Psychotherapy: Co-constructing Interactions.* New Jersey: The Analytic Press.
Solms, M. (2021). *The Hidden Spring: A Journey to the Source of Consciousness.* London. Profile Books.
Tronick, E., Adamson, L.B., Als, H., and Brazelton, T.B. (1975). 'Infant emotions in normal and perturbated interactions'. Paper presented at the biennial meeting of the Society for Research in Child Development, April 1975. Denver, CO.

Introduction

Ainsworth, M.D.S., Blehar, M.C., Waters, E. and Wall, S. (1978). *Patterns of Attachment: A Psychological Study of the Strange Situation.* Hillsdale, NJ: Erlbaum.
Alexander, F. (1950). *Psychosomatic Medicine.* W.W. Norton & Company, Inc. New York.
Beebe, B. and Lachmann, F. (2002). *Infant Research and Adult Psychotherapy: Co-constructing Interactions.* New Jersey: The Analytic Press.
Benjamin, J. (1988). *The Bonds of Love.* Pantheon Books.
Breuer, J. and Freud, S. (1895). *Studies on Hysteria.* S.E. 2., London: Hogarth.
Damasio, A. (1994). *Descartes' Error: Emotion, Reason, and the Human Brain.* New York: Putnam.
Damasio, A. (1999). *The Feeling of What Happens: Body and Emotion in the Making of Consciousness.* New York: Harcourt, Brace & Company.
Ellenberger, H.F. (1970). *The Discovery of the Unconscious.* New York: Basic Books.
Ferenczi, S. (1916–17). 'Disease or patho-neuroses'. In S. Ferenczi, *Further Contributions to the Theory and Technique of Psychoanalysis.* London: Karnac, 1994.
Fonagy, P., Steele, H. and Steele, M. (1991). 'Maternal representations of attachment during pregnancy predict the organisation of infant-mother attachment at one year of age'. *Child Development*, 62, 891–905.
Fordham, M. (1960). 'Countertransference'. In M. Fordham, J. Hubback, R. Gordon and K. Lambert (eds), *Technique in Jungian Analysis.* London: Karnac.

Freud, S. (1895). *Project for a Scientific Psychology. S.E., 1.* London: Hogarth Press.
Freud, S. (1905). *Three Essays on the Theory of Sexuality. S.E., 7.* pp. 125–245. London: Hogarth Press.
Freud, S. (1905b). *Fragment of an Analysis of a Case of Hysteria. S.E., 7.* pp. 7-111. London: Hogarth Press.
Freud, S. (1915a). *Instincts and Their Vicissitudes. S.E., 14.* pp. 109–40. LLondon: Hogarth Press.
Freud, S. (1915b). *The Unconscious. S.E., 14.* pp. 160–215. London: Hogarth Press.
Freud, S. (1923). *The Ego and the Id. S.E., 19.* pp. 3–62. London: Hogarth Press.
Goldberg, P. (2004). 'Fabricated bodies: a model for the somatic false self'. *International Journal of Psycho-Analysis*, 85, 823–40.
Jung, C.G. (1913). The theory of psychoanalysis. *Psychoanalytic Review*, 1(1), 1–40.
Jung, C.G. (1954). *On the Nature of the Psyche. CW8.* London: Routledge & Kegan Paul.
Jung, C.G. (1958). *The Practice of Psychotherapy. CW16.* London: Routledge & Kegan Paul.
Lemma, A. (2010). *Under the Skin: A Psychoanalytic Study of Body Modification.* London and New York: Routledge.
Levine, P. (2015). *Trauma and Memory.* Berkeley, CA: North Atlantic Books.
McDougall, J. (1989). *Theatres of the Body: A Psychoanalytic Approach to Psychosomatic Illness.* New York: Norton.
Main, M. (1991). 'Metacognitive knowledge, metacognitive monitoring, and singular (coherent) vs. multiple (incoherent) models of attachment. findings and directions for future research', in M.C., Parkes, J. Stevenson-Hinde and P. Marris (eds), *Attachment Across the Life Cycle*, Chapter 8. London: Tavistock/Routledge.
Orbach, S. (1978). *Fat is a Feminist Issue.* [Reprinted: Arrow Books, 1998].
Orbach, S. (1986). *Hunger Strike.* [Reprinted: London: Karnac, 2005].
Orbach, S. (2002). 'The true self and the false self'. In B. Kahr (ed.), *The Legacy of Winnicott.* London: Karnac.
Orbach, S. (2009). *Bodies.* London: Profile Books.
Petrucelli, J. (2015). '"My body is a cage": interfacing interpersonal neurobiology, attachment, affect regulation, self-regulation, and the regulation of relatedness in treatment with patients with eating disorders', In J. Petrucelli (ed.), *Body-states: Interpersonal and Relational Perspectives on the Treatment of Eating Disorders.* New York: Routledge.
Schore, A. (1994). *Affect Regulation and the Origin of the Self: The Neurobiology of Emotional Development.* [Reprinted: Routledge, 2016].
Sinason, V. (1992). *Mental Handicap and the Human Condition.* London: Free Association Books.
Solms, M. (2015). *The Feeling Brain.* London: Karnac.
Solms, M. (2021). *The Hidden Spring: A Journey to the Source of Consciousness.* London: Profile Books.
Van der Kolk, B. (2014). *The Body Keeps the Score.* London: Penguin Books.

Williams, G. (1997). *Internal Landscapes and Foreign Bodies*. London: Karnac.
Wooldridge, T. (2018). 'The entropic body: primitive anxieties and secondary skin formation in anorexia nervosa', *Psychoanalytic Dialogues*, 28(2), 189–202.

Chapter 1

Abraham, K. (1907). Letter to Sigmund Freud. 21st December. In S. Freud and K. Abraham (2009). *Briefwechsel 1907–1925: Vollständige Ausgabe. Band 1: 1907–1914*. E. Falzeder and L.M. Hermanns (eds), p. 73. Vienna: Verlag Turia und Kant.
Abraham, K. (1917). 'Über Ejaculatio praecox'. *Internationale Zeitschrift für ärztliche Psychoanalyse*, 4, 171–86.
Abraham, K. (1919). 'Über eine besondere Form des neurotischen Widerstandes gegen die psychoanalytische Methodik'. *Internationale Zeitschrift für ärztliche Psychoanalyse*, 5, 173–80.
Abraham, K. (1920). 'Zur narzißtischen Bewertung der Exkretionsvorgänge in Traum und Neurose'. *Internationale Zeitschrift für Psychoanalyse*, 6, 64–7.
Anderson, R. (1997). 'Putting the boot in: Violent defenses against depressive anxiety'. In R. Schafer (ed.), *The Contemporary Kleinians of London*, pp. 223–38. Madison, Connecticut: International Universities Press.
Anthony, E.J. (1957). 'An experimental approach to the psychopathology of childhood: Encopresis'. *British Journal of Medical Psychology*, 30, 146–75.
Barrows, P. (1996). 'Soiling children: the Oedipal configuration'. *Journal of Child Psychotherapy*, 22, 240–60.
Bick, E. (1964). 'Notes on infant observation in psycho-analytic training'. *International Journal of Psycho-Analysis*, 45, 558–66.
Bion, W.R. (1962a). *Learning from Experience*. London: William Heinemann Medical Books.
Bion, W.R. (1962b). 'The psycho-analytic study of thinking: II. A theory of thinking'. *International Journal of Psycho-Analysis*, 43, 306–10.
Bion, W.R. (1970). *Attention and Interpretation: A Scientific Approach to Insight in Psycho-Analysis and Groups*. London: Tavistock Publications.
Blackman, N. (2003). *Loss and Learning Disability*. London: Worth Publishing.
Breuer, J. (1895). 'Beobachtung I. Frl. Anna O ...'. In J. Breuer and S. Freud. *Studien über Hysterie*, pp. 15–37. Vienna: Franz Deuticke.
Brill, A.A. (1932). 'The sense of smell in the neuroses and psychoses'. *Psychoanalytic Quarterly*, 1, 7–42.
Corbett, A. (2014). *Disabling Perversions: Forensic Psychotherapy with People with Intellectual Disabilities*. London: Karnac Books.
Corbett, A. (2018). 'Extraordinary therapy: On splitting, kindness, and handicapping mothers'. In B. Kahr (ed.). *New Horizons in Forensic Psychotherapy: Exploring the Work of Estela V. Welldon*, pp. 205–18. London: Karnac Books.

Corbett, A., Cottis, T. and Morris, S. (1996). *Witnessing Nurturing Protesting: Therapeutic Responses to Sexual Abuse of People with Learning Disabilities*. London: David Fulton Publishers.

Cottis, T. (2009). 'Life support or intensive care?: Endings and outcomes in psychotherapy for people with intellectual disabilities'. In T. Cottis (ed.), *Intellectual Disability, Trauma and Psychotherapy*, pp. 189–204. London and Hove: Routledge/Taylor and Francis Group.

Cottis, T. (2017). 'You *Can* Take It With You': Transitions and transitional objects in psychotherapy with children who have learning disabilities'. *British Journal of Psychotherapy*, 33, 17–30.

Curen, R. (2009). '"Can They See in the Door?": Issues in the assessment and treatment of sex offenders who have intellectual disabilities'. In T. Cottis (ed.), *Intellectual Disability, Trauma and Psychotherapy*, pp. 90–113. London and Hove: Routledge/Taylor and Francis Group.

Curen, R. (2018). 'Responses to trauma, enactments of trauma: The psychodynamics of an intellectually disabled family'. In B. Kahr (ed.), *New Horizons in Forensic Psychotherapy: Exploring the Work of Estela V. Welldon*, pp. 219–35. London: Karnac Books.

Eder, M. (1924). 'From child life'. *International Journal of Psycho-Analysis*, 5, 201.

Elmhirst, S.I. (1981). 'Bion and babies'. *Annual of Psychoanalysis*, 8, 155–67. New York: International Universities Press.

Elmhirst, S.I. (1996). Personal communication to the author. 25th January.

Fliess, R. (1949). 'Silence and verbalization: A supplement to the theory of the "analytic rule"'. *International Journal of Psycho-Analysis*, 30, 21–30.

Flügel, J.C. (1932). *An Introduction to Psycho-Analysis*. London: Victor Gollancz.

Flynn, D. (1987). 'Internal conflict and growth in a child preparing to start school'. *Journal of Child Psychotherapy*, 13(1), 77–91.

Forsyth, D. (1922). *The Technique of Psycho-Analysis*. London: Kegan Paul, Trench, Trubner and Company.

Forth, M.J. (1992). 'The little-girl lost: Psychotherapy with an anal-retentive and soiling four year old'. *Journal of Child Psychotherapy*, 18(2), 63–85.

Frankish, P. (2016). *Disability Psychotherapy: An Innovative Approach to Trauma-Informed Care*. London: Karnac Books.

Freud, S. (1900a). *Die Traumdeutung*. Vienna: Franz Deuticke.

Freud, S. (1900b). *The Interpretation of Dreams*. J. Strachey (trans.). In S. Freud (1953) *The Standard Edition of the Complete Psychological Works of Sigmund Freud: Volume IV. (1900). The Interpretation of Dreams. (First Part)*. J. Strachey, A. Freud, A. Strachey and A. Tyson (eds. and trans.), pp. xxiii–338. London: Hogarth Press and the Institute of Psycho-Analysis.

Freud, S. (1900c). *The Interpretation of Dreams*. J. Strachey (trans.). In S. Freud (1953) *The Standard Edition of the Complete Psychological Works of Sigmund Freud: Volume V. (1900-1901). The Interpretation of Dreams. (Second Part) and On Dreams*. J. Strachey, A. Freud, A. Strachey and A. Tyson

(eds. and trans.), pp. 339-621. London: Hogarth Press and the Institute of Psycho-Analysis.
Freud, S. (1905). *Drei Abhandlungen zur Sexualtheorie*. Vienna: Franz Deuticke.
Freud, S. (1906a). Letter to Carl Gustav Jung. 27th October. In S. Freud and C.G. Jung (1974). *Briefwechsel*. W. McGuire and W. Sauerländer (eds.), pp. 8-9. Frankfurt am Main: S. Fischer/S. Fischer Verlag.
Freud, S. (1906b). Letter to Carl Gustav Jung. 27th October. In S. Freud and C.G. Jung (1974). *The Freud/Jung Letters: The Correspondence Between Sigmund Freud and C.G. Jung*. W. McGuire (ed.) R. Manheim and R.F.C. Hull (trans.), pp. 8-9. Princeton, New Jersey: Princeton University Press.
Freud, S. (1907). Letter to Carl Gustav Jung. 14th April. In S. Freud and C.G. Jung (1974). *Briefwechsel*. W. McGuire and W. Sauerländer (eds.), pp. 35-38. Frankfurt am Main: S. Fischer/S. Fischer Verlag.
Freud, S. (1908a). Letter to Karl Abraham. 1st January. In S. Freud and K. Abraham (2009). *Briefwechsel 1907-1925: Vollständige Ausgabe. Band 1: 1907-1914*. E. Falzeder and L.M. Hermanns (eds.), p. 75. Vienna: Verlag Turia und Kant.
Freud, S. (1908b). Letter to Karl Abraham. 1st January. In S. Freud and K. Abraham (2002). *The Complete Correspondence of Sigmund Freud and Karl Abraham: 1907-1925. Completed Edition*. E. Falzeder (ed.), C. Schwarzacher, C. Trollope and K.M. King (trans.), p. 16. London: H. Karnac (Books)/Other Press.
Freud, S. (1909a). 'Analyse der Phobie eines 5jährigen Knaben'. *Jahrbuch für psychoanalytische und psychopathologische Forschungen*, 1, 1-109.
Freud, S. (1909b). 'Bemerkungen über einen Fall von Zwangsneurose'. *Jahrbuch für psychoanalytische und psychopathologische Forschungen*, 1, 357-421.
Freud, S. (1924). Letter to Max Eitingon. 7th October. In S. Freud and M. Eitingon (2004). *Briefwechsel: 1906-1939. Erster Band*. M. Schröter (ed.), pp. 361-3. Tübingen: edition diskord.
Fromm-Reichmann, F. (1935). Process Notes. 29th July, 1935 – 25th August, 1935. Chestnut Lodge Archive, Rockville, Maryland, USA. Cited in G.A. Hornstein (2000). *To Redeem One Person is to Redeem the World: The Life of Frieda Fromm-Reichmann*, p. 415, n. 53. New York: Free Press/Simon and Schuster.
Fromm-Reichmann, F. (1948). 'Notes on the development of treatment of schizophrenics by psychoanalytic psychotherapy'. *Psychiatry*, 11, 263-73.
Fromm-Reichmann, F. (1954). 'Psychotherapy of schizophrenia'. *American Journal of Psychiatry*, 111, 410-19.
Harris, M. (1987). Papers on infant observation. In M.P.H. Williams (ed.), *The Collected Papers of Martha Harris and Esther Bick*, pp. 219-39. Strath Tay, Perthshire, Scotland: Clunie Press.
Hinshelwood, R.D. (1989). *A Dictionary of Kleinian Thought*. London: Free Association Books.
Hinshelwood, R.D. (1994). *Clinical Klein*. London: Free Association Books.
Hollins, S. (1997). 'Counselling and psychotherapy'. In O. Russell (ed.), *Seminars*

in the *Psychiatry of Learning Disabilities*, pp. 245-58. London: Gaskell/Royal College of Psychiatrists.

Hollins, S. (2002). 'What is the future of the psychiatry of learning disability?' *Psychiatric Bulletin: The Journal of Psychiatric Practice*, 26, 283-4.

Hollins, S. and Sinason, V. (2000). 'Psychotherapy, learning disabilities and trauma: New perspectives'. *British Journal of Psychiatry*, 176, 32-36.

Jones, E. (1922). Letter to Sigmund Freud. 22nd January. In S. Freud and E. Jones (1993). *The Complete Correspondence of Sigmund Freud and Ernest Jones: 1908-1939*. R.A. Paskauskas (ed.), pp. 453-4. Cambridge, Massachusetts: Belknap Press of Harvard University Press.

Jones, E. (1955). *The Life and Work of Sigmund Freud: Volume 2. Years of Maturity. 1901-1919*. New York: Basic Books.

Jones, E. (1957). *The Life and Work of Sigmund Freud: Volume 3. The Last Phase. 1919-1939*. New York: Basic Books.

Jung, C.G. (1906a). Letter to Sigmund Freud. 23rd October. In S. Freud and C.G. Jung (1974). *Briefwechsel*. W. McGuire and W. Sauerländer (eds), pp. 6-7. Frankfurt am Main: S. Fischer/S. Fischer Verlag.

Jung, C.G. (1906b). Letter to Sigmund Freud. 23rd October. In S. Freud and C.G. Jung (1974). *The Freud/Jung Letters: The Correspondence Between Sigmund Freud and C.G. Jung*. W. McGuire (ed.), R. Manheim and R.F.C. Hull (trans.), pp. 6-7. Princeton, New Jersey: Princeton University Press.

Jung, C.G. (1907a). Letter to Sigmund Freud. 17th April. In S. Freud and C.G. Jung (1974). *Briefwechsel*. W. McGuire and W. Sauerländer (eds.), pp. 39-41. Frankfurt am Main: S. Fischer/S. Fischer Verlag.

Jung, C.G. (1907b). Letter to Sigmund Freud. 13th May. In S. Freud and C.G. Jung (1974). *Briefwechsel*. W. McGuire and W. Sauerländer (eds.), pp. 47-50. Frankfurt am Main: S. Fischer/S. Fischer Verlag.

Jung, C.G. (1907c). Letter to Sigmund Freud. 12th June. In S. Freud and C.G. Jung (1974). *Briefwechsel*. W. McGuire and W. Sauerländer (eds.), pp. 68-70. Frankfurt am Main: S. Fischer/S. Fischer Verlag.

Kahr, B. (1994). Telephone interview with Frances Tustin. 22nd February.

Kahr, B. (1995). Lecture on 'Mucus, Saliva, Urine, Faeces, Semen, Menstrual Blood, Flatus, Vomitus, and Phlegm: On Patients Who Evacuate Bodily Fluids in Psychotherapy'. Tavistock Clinic Mental Handicap Workshop. Child and Family Department, Tavistock Clinic, Tavistock Centre, Tavistock and Portman NHS Trust, Belsize Park, London. 16th June.

Kahr, B. (1996). Lecture on 'The Escorted Treatment'. Open Meeting, Tavistock Clinic Mental Handicap Workshop. Child and Family Department, Tavistock Clinic, Tavistock Centre, Tavistock and Portman NHS Trust, Belsize Park, London. 4th November.

Kahr, B. (1997). Lecture on 'Patients Who Evacuate Bodily Fluids During Psychotherapy'. Tavistock Clinic Mental Handicap Workshop. Child and Family Department, Tavistock Clinic, Tavistock Centre, Tavistock and

Portman NHS Trust, Belsize Park, London. 10th November.
Kahr, B. (2005). 'On patients who remove their clothing in sessions'. *American Imago*, 62, 217–23.
Kahr, B. (2008). 'Tissues'. *American Imago*, 65, 299–308.
Kahr, B. (2012). 'The infanticidal origins of psychosis: The role of trauma in schizophrenia'. In J. Yellin and K. White (eds.), *Shattered States: Disorganized Attachment and its Repair. The John Bowlby Memorial Conference Monograph 2007*, pp. 7–126. London: Karnac Books.
Kahr, B. (2017). 'From the treatment of a compulsive spitter: A psychoanalytical approach to profound disability'. *British Journal of Psychotherapy*, 33, 31–47.
Kahr B. (2019). '"Slashing the teddy bear's tummy with a carving knife": The infanticidal roots of schizophrenia'. *British Journal of Psychotherapy*, 35, 399–416.
Kahr, B. (2020a). *Bombs in the Consulting Room: Surviving Psychological Shrapnel*. London and Abingdon, Oxfordshire: Routledge/Taylor and Francis Group.
Kahr, B. (2020b). *On Practising Therapy at 1.45 A.M.: Adventures of a Clinician*. London and Abingdon, Oxfordshire: Routledge/Taylor and Francis Group.
Kahr, B. (2021a). 'Insults and spears: The tribulations of forensic disability psychotherapy'. In N. Beail, P. Frankish and A. Skelly (eds), *Trauma and Intellectual Disability: Acknowledgement, Identification and Intervention*, pp. 175–88. Shoreham by Sea, West Sussex: Pavilion/Pavilion Publishing and Media.
Kahr, B. (2021b). 'Mucus, saliva, urine, and menstrual blood: On patients who evacuate bodily fluids in psychotherapy'. *Body, Movement and Dance in Psychotherapy*, 16, 230–43.
Kahr, B. (2021c). 'On patients who explode: Surviving petrifying psychotherapeutic experiences'. *International Journal of Forensic Psychotherapy*, 3, 93-112.
Kardiner, A. (1977). *My Analysis with Freud: Reminiscences*. New York: W.W. Norton and Company.
Kerr, J. (1993). *A Most Dangerous Method: The Story of Jung, Freud, and Sabina Spielrein*. New York: Alfred A. Knopf.
Khan, M.M.R. (1963). 'Silence as communication'. *Bulletin of the Menninger Clinic*, 27, 300–13.
Klein, M. (1932). *Die Psychoanalyse des Kindes*. Vienna: Internationaler Psychoanalytischer Verlag.
Klein, M. (1935). 'A contribution to the psychogenesis of manic-depressive states'. *International Journal of Psycho-Analysis*, 16, 145–74.
Klein, M. (1946). 'Notes on some schizoid mechanisms'. *International Journal of Psycho-Analysis*, 27, 99–110.
Kraepelin, E. (1913). *Psychiatrie: Ein Lehrbuch für Studierende und Ärzte. Achte, vollständig umgearbeitete Auflage. III. Band. Klinische Psychiatrie. II. Teil*. Leipzig: Verlag von Johann Ambrosius Barth.
Langs, R. (1973). *The Technique of Psychoanalytic Psychotherapy: Volume I. The Initial Contact. Theoretical Framework. Understanding the Patient's*

Communications. The Therapist's Interventions. New York: Jason Aronson.
Launer, J. (2014). *Sex Versus Survival: The Life and Ideas of Sabina Spielrein*. London: Duckworth Overlook.
Lewin, B.D. (1930). 'Kotschmieren, Menses und weibliches Über-Ich'. *Internationale Zeitschrift für Psychoanalyse*, 16, 43–56.
Miller, L. (1999). 'Infant observation as a precursor of clinical training'. *Psychoanalytic Inquiry*, 19, 142–5.
Money-Kyrle, R. (1971). 'The aim of psychoanalysis'. *International Journal of Psycho-Analysis*, 52, 103–6.
Richebächer, S. (2005). *Sabina Spielrein: 'Eine fast grausame Liebe zur Wissenschaft'*. Zürich: Dörlemann/Dörlemann Verlag.
Roazen, P. (1969). *Brother Animal: The Story of Freud and Tausk*. New York: Alfred A. Knopf.
Roazen, P. (1995). *How Freud Worked: First-Hand Accounts of Patients*. Northvale, New Jersey: Jason Aronson.
Rosenfeld, S. (1968). 'Choice of symptom: Notes on a case of retention'. *Journal of Child Psychotherapy*, 2(2), 38–49.
Rosenfeld, H. (1987). *Impasse and Interpretation: Therapeutic and Anti-Therapeutic Factors in the Psychoanalytic Treatment of Psychotic, Borderline, and Neurotic Patients*. London: Tavistock Publications.
Rustin, M. (1989). 'Encountering primitive anxieties'. In L. Miller, M. Rustin, M. Rustin and J. Shuttleworth (eds.), *Closely Observed Infants*, pp. 7–21. London: Gerald Duckworth and Company.
Scharff, J.S. and Scharff, D.E. (1992). *Scharff Notes: A Primer of Object Relations Therapy*. Northvale, New Jersey: Jason Aronson.
Schick, A. (1948). 'A case of psychogenic vomiting'. *American Journal of Psychotherapy*, 2, 108–13.
Shane, M. (1967). 'Encopresis in a latency boy. An arrest along a developmental line'. *Psychoanalytic Study of the Child*, 22, 296–314. New York: International Universities Press.
Sinason, V. (1986). 'Secondary mental handicap and its relationship to trauma'. *Psychoanalytic Psychotherapy*, 2, 131–54.
Sinason, V. (1988). 'Smiling, swallowing, sickening and stupefying: The effect of sexual abuse on the child'. *Psychoanalytic Psychotherapy*, 3, 97–111.
Sinason, V. (1991). 'Interpretations that feel horrible to make and a theoretical unicorn'. *Journal of Child Psychotherapy*, 17, 11–24.
Sinason, V. (1992). *Mental Handicap and the Human Condition: New Approaches from the Tavistock*. London: Free Association Books.
Sinason, V. (1999). 'Psychoanalysis and mental handicap: Experience from the Tavistock Clinic'. In J. De Groef and E. Heinemann (eds.), *Psychoanalysis and Mental Handicap*. A. Weller (trans.), pp. 194–206. London: Free Association Books.
Sinason, V. (2012). 'Infanticide and paedophilia as a defence against incest: Work with a man with a severe intellectual disability'. In J. Adlam, A. Aiyegbusi, P.

Kleinot, A. Motz and C. Scanlon (eds.), *The Therapeutic Milieu Under Fire: Security and Insecurity in Forensic Mental Health*, pp. 175–85. London: Jessica Kingsley Publishers.
Socarides, C.W. (1969). 'Psychoanalytic therapy of a male homosexual'. *Psychoanalytic Quarterly*, 38, 173–90.
Sterba, E. (1934). 'Aus der Analyse eines Zweijährigen'. *Zeitschrift für psychoanalytische Pädagogik*, 8, 37–72.
Strachey, J. (1934). 'The nature of the therapeutic action of psycho-analysis'. *International Journal of Psycho-Analysis*, 15, 127–59.
Tirelli, L.C. (1989). 'Some observations on the relationship between language and verbal thought in a psychotic adolescent'. *Journal of Child Psychotherapy*, 15(1), 113–25.
Tustin, F. (1981). *Autistic States in Children*. London: Routledge and Kegan Paul.
Tustin, F. (1986). *Autistic Barriers in Neurotic Patients*. London: H. Karnac (Books).
Weininger, B.I. (1989). 'Chestnut Lodge – The early years: Krishnamurti and Buber'. In A-L.S. Silver (ed.), *Psychoanalysis and Psychosis*, pp. 495–512. Madison, Connecticut: International Universities Press.
Wilson, S. (2003). *Disability, Counselling and Psychotherapy: Challenges and Opportunities*. Houndmills, Basingstoke, Hampshire: Palgrave Macmillan.
Winnicott, D.W. (1941). 'The Observation of Infants in a Set Situation'. *International Journal of Psycho-Analysis*, 22, 229–49.
Winnicott, D.W. (1962). 'The aims of psycho-analytical treatment'. In D.W. Winnicott (1965). *The Maturational Processes and the Facilitating Environment: Studies in the Theory of Emotional Development*, pp. 166–70. London: Hogarth Press and the Institute of Psycho-Analysis.
Winnicott, D.W. (1963). 'Communicating and not communicating leading to a study of certain opposites'. In D.W. Winnicott (1965). *The Maturational Processes and the Facilitating Environment: Studies in the Theory of Emotional Development*, pp. 179–92. London: Hogarth Press and the Institute of Psycho-Analysis.
Winnicott, D.W. (1969). 'The use of an object'. *International Journal of Psycho-Analysis*, 50, 711–16.

Chapter 2

Sinason, V. (1995). *Night Shift: New Poems*. London: Karnac.
Sinason, V. (2010). *Mental Handicap and the Human Condition: An Analytic Approach to Intellectual Disability*. London: Free Association Books.

Chapter 3

Brown, H, Stein J, Tuck, V. (1995). The sexual abuse of adults with learning disabilities: Report of a second two-year incidence survey. *Mental Handicap Research*, 8(1) 22-24.

Cooper, S.A., Smiley, E., Morrison, J., Williamson, A. and Allan, L. (2007). 'Mental ill-health in adults with intellectual disabilities: prevalence and associated factors'. *British Journal of Psychiatry*, 190, 27–35.

Corbett, A. (2014). *Disabling Perversions*. London: Karnac.

Corbett, A. (2019). *Intellectual Disability and Psychotherapy: the Theories, Practice and Influence of Valerie Sinason*. Abingdon: Routledge.

Cottis, T. (ed.) (2008). *Intellectual Disability, Trauma and Psychotherapy*. London: Routledge.

Cottis, T. (2019). 'We are who we see looking back at us: Valerie as a supporter of a developing organisation'. In A. Corbett (2019). *Intellectual Disability and Psychotherapy: the Theories, Practice and Influence of Valerie Sinason*. Abingdon: Routledge.

Cottis, T. and O'Driscoll, D. (2009). 'Outside In: The effects of trauma on organisations'. In T. Cottis (ed.), *Intellectual Disability, Trauma and Psychotherapy*. London: Routledge.

Dodd, P., Guerin, S., McEvoy, J., Buckley, S., Tyrrell, J. and Hillery, J. (2008). 'A study of complicated grief symptoms in people with intellectual disabilities'. *Journal of Intellectual Disability Research*, 52(5), 415–25.

Heslop, P. and Lovell, A. (2013). *Understanding and Working with People with Learning Disabilities who Self-injure*. London: Jessica Kingsley.

Heslop, P. and Macaulay, F. (2009). *Hidden Pain? Self-Injury and People with Learning Disabilities*. Bristol: Bristol Crisis Service for Women.

Hodges, S. (2003). *Counselling Adults with Learning Disabilities*. New York. Palgrave. Macmillan.

Hollins, S., Dowling, S. and Blackman, N. (2003). *When Somebody Dies*. London: Books Beyond Words.

Hollins, S. and Sireling, L. (2004). *When Mum Died*. London: Books Beyond Words.

Jarrett. S. (2020). *Those They Called Idiots. The Idea of the Disabled Mind From 1700 to the Present Day*. London: Reaktion Books.

Kahr, B. (2000). 'The adventures of a psychotherapist: a new breed of clinicians – disability psychotherapists'. *Psychotherapy Review*, 2, 193–4.

Kahr, B. (2017). 'From the treatment of a compulsive spitter: A psychoanalytical approach to profound disability'. *British Journal of Psychotherapy*, 33, 31–47.

Keats, J. (1817). *Letters*. Oxford: Oxford University Press.

Levitas, A.S. and Hurley, A.D. (2007). 'Overmedication as a manifestation of countertransference'. *Mental Health Aspects of Developmental Disabilities*, 10(2), 1–5.

NHS England. *Stopping Over Medication of People with a Learning Disability, Autism or Both* (STOMP). London: NHS England (undated). www.england.nhs.uk/learning-disabilities/improving-health/stomp/

O'Driscoll, D. (2014). 'In a better place? How far we have come in addressing service users grief and sense of loss following bereavement'. *Learning Disability Practice* 17(8), 13.

O'Driscoll, D. (2015). 'Anti-hate crime'. In B. Gates, D. Fearns and J. Welch (eds.), *Learning Disability Nursing at a Glance*. Chichester: Wiley Blackwell.

O'Driscoll, D. (2018). 'Facing the final curtain'. *Learning Disability Practice*, 21(3), 13.

O'Driscoll D. (2019). 'Building insight and changing lives: the contribution of Valerie Sinason to the history of disability psychotherapy'. In A. Corbett (2019) *Intellectual Disability and Psychotherapy: the Theories, Practice and Influence of Valerie Sinason*. pp 93–105. Abingdon: Routledge.

Parsons, J. and Upton, P. (1986). *Psychodynamic psychotherapy with mentally handicapped patients: technical issues*. Tavistock paper 3, unpublished paper.

Phelvin, A. (2012). 'Getting the message: intuition and reflexivity in professional interpretations of non-verbal behaviours in people with profound learning disabilities'. *British Journal of Learning Disabilities*, 41, 31–7.

Shepherd, C. and Beail, N. (2017). 'A systematic review of the effectiveness of psychoanalysis, psychoanalytic and psychodynamic psychotherapy with adults with intellectual and developmental disabilities: progress and challenges'. *Psychoanalytic Psychotherapy*, 31(1), 94–117.

Sinason, V. (1992). *Mental Handicap and The Human Condition: New Approaches From The Tavistock*. London: Free Association Books.

Symington, N. (1981). 'The psychotherapy of a subnormal patient'. *British Journal of Medical Psychology*, 44, 187-199.

Trent, J. (1994). *Inventing the Feeble Mind: A History of Mental Retardation in America*. Berkley: University of California Press.

Wilson, S. (2002). *Disability, Counselling and Psychotherapy. Challenges and Opportunities*. London: Palgrave Macmillan.

Chapter 4

Adlam, J. and Scanlon, C. (2009). 'Disturbances of "groupishness"? Structural violence, refusal and the therapeutic community response to severe personality disorder'. *International Forum of Psychoanalysis*, 18(1), 23–9.

American Psychiatric Association (APA) (2013). *Diagnostic and Statistical Manual* 5th edn. Washington, DC: APA.

Anzieu, D. (1996 [1985]). *The Skin-Ego*. N. Segal (trans.). London: Karnac.

Ashenburg, K. (2007). *Clean: An Unsanitized History of Washing*. London: Profile.

Baez, J. (1975). 'Diamonds and Rust'. Los Angeles: A & M Records.

Bauman, Z. (2004). *Wasted Lives*. Cambridge: Polity Press.

Behr, H. and Hearst, L. (2005). *Group-analytic Psychotherapy: A Meeting of Minds*. London: Whurr.
Bion, W.R. (1961). *Experiences in Groups*. London: Routledge.
Bion, W.R. (2007 [1962]). 'A theory of thinking'. In W.R. Bion *Second Thoughts*, pp. 110–19. London: Karnac.
Borossa, J. (2001). *Hysteria*. Cambridge: Icon Books.
Bourke, J. (2005). *Fear: A Cultural History*. London: Virago.
Brenman Pick, I. (1985). 'Working through in the countertransference'. *International Journal of Psycho-Analysis*, 66, 157–66.
Breuer, J. and Freud, S. (1895). *Studies on Hysteria*. S.E. 2., London: Hogarth.
Brill, A.A. (1932). 'The sense of smell in the neuroses and psychoses'. *Psychoanalytic Quarterly*, 1, 7–42.
Brown, G. (2013). 'On loneliness'. In C. Driver, S. Crawford and J. Stewart (eds) *Being and Relating in Psychotherapy*, pp. 92–106. London: Palgrave Macmillan.
Campbell, J.M. (2019). 'There's no place like home': On dwelling and *Unheimlichkeit*'. In G. Brown (ed.), *Psychoanalytic Thinking on the Unhoused Mind*, pp. 19–35. Abingdon: Routledge.
Chadwick, E. (1842). *Report on an Enquiry into the Sanitary Conditions and the Labouring Population of Great Britain*. London: William Clowes.
Cobb, M. (2020). *Smell: A Very Short Introduction*. Oxford: Oxford University Press.
Cockayne, E. (2007). *Hubbub, Filth, Noise and Stench in England 1600–1700*. London: Yale University Press.
Corbin, A. (1986 [1982]). *The Foul and the Fragrant: Odour and the French Social Imagination*. M. Kochan (trans.). London: Berg.
Cox, R. et al. (2011). *Dirt: The Filthy Reality of Everyday Life*. London: Wellcome.
Douglas, M. (1966). *Purity and Danger*. London: Routledge & Kegan Paul.
Fairbairn, W.R.D. (2006 [1943]). 'The repression and the return of bad objects'. In *Psychoanalytic Studies of the Personality*, pp. 59–81. London: Routledge.
Freud, S. (1905). *Three Essays on the Theory of Sexuality*. S.E., 7. London: Hogarth Press.
Freud, S. (1917). *Mourning and Melancholia*. S.E., 14. London: Hogarth Press.
Freud, S. (1920). *Beyond the Pleasure Principle*. S.E., 18. pp. 1–64. London: Hogarth Press.
Freud, S. (1923). *The Ego and the Id*. S.E., 19. pp. 1–66. London: Hogarth Press.
Freud, S. (1930). *Civilization and Its Discontents*. S.E., 21. pp. 57–145. London: Hogarth Press.
Freud, S. (1961). *Letters of Sigmund Freud 1873–1939*. E.L. Freud (ed.), T. and J. Stern (trans.). London: Hogarth Press.
Freud, S. (1985). *The Complete Letters of Sigmund Freud to Wilhelm Fliess 1887–1904*. J.M. Masson (trans. and ed.). Cambridge, MA: Harvard University Press.
Friedman, P. (1959). 'Some observations on the sense of smell'. *Psychoanalytic Quarterly*, 28, 307–29.

Fryer, P. (1984/2018). *Staying Power: The History of Black People in Britain*. London: Pluto Press.

Gardner, F. (1999). 'A sense of all conditions'. In D. Mann (ed.), *Erotic Transference and Countertransference*, pp. 139–49. London: Routledge.

Geller, J. (2011). *The Other Jewish Question: Identifying the Jew and Making Sense of Modernity*. New York: Fordham University Press.

Gilligan, J. (1996). *Violence: Reflections on our Deadliest Epidemic*. London: Jessica Kingsley.

Hall, S. (2018). *Familiar Stranger: A Life Between Two Islands*. London: Penguin Books.

Hempel, S. (2006). *The Medical Detective: John Snow, Cholera and the Broad Street Pump*. London: Granta.

Jenner, M. (2000). 'Civilization and deodorization? Smell in early modern English culture'. In P. Burke et al. (eds.), *Civil Histories: Essays Presented to Sir Keith Thomas*, pp. 127–44. Oxford: Oxford University Press.

Jenner, M.S.R. (2011). 'Follow your nose? Smell, smelling, and their histories'. *American Historical Review*, 116(2), 335–51.

Kettler, A. (2020). *The Smell of Slavery: Olfactory Racism and the Atlantic World*. Cambridge: Cambridge University Press.

Klein, M. (1993 [1959]). 'Our adult world and its roots in infancy'. In M. Klein *Envy and Gratitude and Other Works 1946–1963*, pp. 247–63. London: Virago.

Klein, M. (1993 [1963]). 'On the sense of loneliness'. In M. Klein *Envy and Gratitude and Other Works 1946–1963*, pp. 300–13. London: Virago.

Lagerspetz, O. (2018). *A Philosophy of Dirt*. London: Reaktion Books.

Lemma, A. (2010). *Under the Skin: A Psychoanalytic Study of Body Modification*. London: Routledge.

Lemma, A. (2015) *Minding the Body: The Body in Psychoanalysis and Beyond*. East Sussex: Routledge.

Menninghaus, W. (2003). *Disgust: Theory and History of a Strong Sensation*. Albany: State University of New York Press.

Miller, S. (2004). *Disgust: The Gatekeeper of Emotion*. Hillsdale, NJ: The Analytic Press.

Mollon, P. (1993). *The Fragile Self*. London: Whurr.

Mollon, P. (2005). 'The inherent shame of sexuality'. *British Journal of Psychotherapy*, 22(2), 167–78.

Naphy, W. and Roberts, P. (1997). *Fear in Early Modern Society*. Manchester: Manchester University Press.

NICE (2009). Child maltreatment: when to suspect maltreatment in under 18s Clinical guideline [CG89]. www.nice.org.uk/nicemedia/pdf/CG89FullGuideline.pdf. Accessed 31 January 2022.

Nussbaum, N.C. (1999). 'Secret sewers of vice'. In S. Bandes (ed.), *The Passions of Law*. New York: New York University Press.

Oxford Dictionaries (2018a). s.v. Communicate. In *Oxford Dictionary of English*. Oxford: Oxford University Press.

Oxford Dictionaries (2018b). s.v. Hygiene. In *Oxford Dictionary of English*. Oxford: Oxford University Press.
Peto, A. (1973). 'The olfactory forerunner of the superego: Its role in normalcy, neurosis and fetishism'. *International Journal of Psycho-Analysis*, 54, 323–30.
Rosenfeld, H. (1960). *Psychotic States. A Psychoanalytic Approach*. London. Hogarth Press.
Scanlon, C. and Adlam, J. (2019). 'Housing un-housed minds: Complex multiple exclusion and the cycle of rejection revisited'. In G. Brown (ed.), *Psychoanalytic Thinking on the Unhoused Mind*, pp. 1–18. Abingdon: Routledge.
Segal, H. (1997). 'Termination: Sweating it out'. In H. Segal *Psychoanalysis, Literature and War: Papers 1972-1995*, pp. 103–10. London: Routledge.
Sidoli, M. (1996). 'Farting as a defence against unspeakable dread'. *Analytical Psychology*, 41(2), 165–78.
Spector, T. (2015). *The Diet Myth*. London: Weidenfeld & Nicolson.
Stallybrass, P. and White, A. (1986). *The Politics and Poetics of Transgression*. London: Methuen.
Stekel, W. (1967 [1910]). 'Symposium on suicide'. In P. Friedman (ed.), *On Suicide: With Particular Reference to Suicide Among Young Students*, pp. 33–141. New York: International Universities Press.
Winnicott, D.W. (1990 [1960]). 'The Theory of the Parent-Infant Relationship'. In D.W. Winnicott *The Maturational Process and the Facilitating Environment*, pp. 37–55. London: Karnac.
Winnicott, D.W. (1974). 'Fear of Breakdown'. *International Review of Psycho-Analysis*, 1, 103–7.

Chapter 5

Anzieu, D. (1995). *The Skin-Ego*. London: Karnac.
Bick, E. (1968). 'The experience of the skin in early object-relations'. *International Journal of Psychoanalysis*, 49(2-3), 484–6.
Bick, E. (1986). 'Further considerations on the function of the skin in early object-relations'. *British Journal of Psychotherapy*, 2, 292–9.
Bion, W.R. (1959). '*Attacks on linking*'. *International Journal of Psycho-Analysis*, 40, 308–15.
Bion, W.R. (1962). 'A theory of thinking'. *International Journal of Psycho-Analysis*, 43, 306–10.
Britton, R. (2003). *Sex, Death and the Superego*. London & New York: Karnac.
Brown, G. (2015). 'Psychotherapy with people who smell'. *Psychoanalysis, Culture & Society*, 20(1), 29–48.
Glasser, M. (1979). 'Some aspects of the role of aggression in the perversions'. In I. Rosen (ed.), *Sexual Deviations*, pp. 278–305. Oxford: Oxford University Press.
Kahr, B. (2007). 'The infanticidal origins of psychosis'. *Attachment: New Directions*

in Psychotherapy and Relational Psychoanalysis, 1, 117–32.
Klein, M. (1932). *The Psycho-Analysis of Children*. London: Hogarth Press.
Meltzer, D. (1992). *The Claustrum: An Investigation of Claustrophobic Phenomena*. Perthshire: Clunie Press.
Mitrani, J.L. (1995). 'On adhesive pseudo-object relations: II. Illustration'. *Contemporary Psychoanalysis*, 31(1), 140.
Nabokov, V. (1970). *Mary*. Reprinted 2007. London: Penguin Books.
O'Shaughnessy, E. (2015). *Inquiries in Psychoanalysis: Collected Papers of Edna O'Shaughnessy*. London: Routledge.
Odgen, T. (1989). *The Primitive Edge of Experience*. Reprinted 2018, London and New York: Routledge.
Proust, M. (1913). *Remembrance of Things Past: 1*. Reprinted 1989, London: Penguin Books.
Sandler, J. (1976). 'Countertransference and role responsiveness'. *International Review of Psycho-Analysis*, 3, 43–7.
Schore, A. (2003). *Affect Disregulation and the Disorders of the Self*. New York: Norton.
Steiner, J. (1993). *Psychic Retreats: Pathological Organizations in Psychotic, Neurotic and Borderline Patients*. London: Routledge.
Stern, D. et al (1998). 'Non-interpretative mechanisms in psychoanalytic therapy. The "something more" than interpretation'. *International Journal of Psychoanalysis*, 79, 903–21.
Strachey, J. (1934). 'The nature of the therapeutic action in psychoanalysis'. *International Journal of Psycho-Analysis*, 15, 127–59.
Süskind, P. (1986). *Perfume: The Story of a Murderer*. Penguin Group.
Winnicott, D.W. (1949). 'Hate in the counter-transference'. *International Journal of Psycho-Analysis*, 30, 69–74.
Winnicott, D.W. (1956). 'Primary Maternal Preoccupation'. In D.W. Winnicott (1958) *Collected Papers: Through Paediatrics to Psychoanalysis*. London: Tavistock Publications.
Winnicott, D.W. (1969). 'The use of an object'. *International Journal of Psycho-Analysis*, 50, 711–16.
Winnicott, D.W. (1971). *Playing and Reality*. London: Tavistock Publications.

Chapter 6

Addison A. (2019). *Jung's Psychoid Concept Contextualized*. Abingdon, Oxon: Routledge.
Bick, E. (1968). 'The experience of the skin in early object-relations'. *International Journal of Psychoanalysis*, 49(2–3), 484–6.
Bion, W.R. (1959). 'Attacks on linking'. *International Journal of Psycho-Analysis*, 40, 308–15.
Bion, W.R. (1962). 'The psycho-analytic study of thinking: II. A theory of thinking'.

International Journal of Psycho-Analysis, 43, 306–10.
Bott Spillius, E. (ed.) (1988). *Melanie Klein Today, Volume 1: Mainly Theory*. London: Routledge.
Callieri, B. (2007). *Corpo, Esistenze, Mondi*. Rome: Edizioni Universitarie Romane.
Caretti, V. (2006). 'La solitudine del curante, la scissione mente-corpo e il deficit della simbolizzazione'. In L. Aversa (ed.), *Simbolo, Metafora, Esistenza. Saggi in Onore di Mario Trevi*, pp. 27–35. Bergamo: Moretti and Vitali.
Carvalho, R. (2014). 'Synchronicity, the infinite unrepressed, dissociation and the interpersonal'. *Journal of Analytical Psychology*, 59(3), 366–84.
Cavalli, A. (2020). 'Noah's Ark: technical and theoretical implications concerning the use of metaphor in treatment of trauma'. *Journal of Analytical Psychology*, 65(5), 780–962.
Clark, G. (1996). 'The animating body: psychoid substance as a mutual experience of psychosomatic disorder'. *Journal of Analytical Psychology*, 41, 353–68.
Connolly, A. (2013). 'Out of the body: embodiment and its vicissitudes'. *Journal of Analytical Psychology*, 58(5), 636–56.
Corbin, H. (1972). *Mundus Imaginalis, or the Imaginary and the Imaginal*. R. Honorine (trans.). Ipswich: Golgonooza Press, 1976.
Corsa, R. and Monterosa, L. (2015). *Limite è Speranza*. Roma: Alpes.
De Rienzo, A. (2021). 'The day the clock stopped. Primitive states of unintegration, multidimensional working through and the birth of the analytical subject'. *Journal of Analytical Psychology*, 67(1), 259–80.
Devescovi, P. C. (2009). 'Aspetti transferali e controtransferali del sonno dell'analista in seduta'. *Studi Junghiani*, 29, 51–69.
Eulert-Fuchs, D. (2020). 'The other between fear and desire – countertransference fantasy as a bridge between me and the other'. *Journal of Analytical Psychology*, 65(1), 153–70.
Ferro, A. (2003). 'Marcella: The transition from explosive sensoriality to the ability to think'. *The Psychoanalytic Quarterly*, 75, 477–500.
Field N. (1989). Listening with the body: An exploration of the countertransference. *British Journal of Psychotherapy*, 5, 512–22
Fordham, M. (1960). 'Countertransference'. In M. Fordham, R. Gordon, J. Hubback and K. Lambert (eds.), *Technique in Jungian Analysis*. London: Karnac, 1989.
Fordham, M. (1969). *Children as Individuals*. New York: C.G. Jung Foundation.
Fordham, M. (1991). 'The supposed limit of interpretation'. *Journal of Analytical Psychology*, 36, 165–75.
Godsil, G. (2018). 'Residues in the analyst of the patient's symbiotic connection at a somatic level: unrepresented states in the patient and analyst'. *Journal of Analytical Psychology*, 63(1), 6–25.
Gordon, R. (1965). 'The concept of projective identification'. *Journal of Analytical Psychology*, 10(2), 127–49.
Grotstein, J.S. (1981). *Splitting and Projective Identification*. New York: Jason Aronson.

References

Hilty, R. (2020). 'Unpleasant bodily odour in a psychoanalytic treatment: bridge or drawbridge to a troubled past'. *British Journal of Psychotherapy*, 36, 200–15.
Joseph, B. (1987). 'Projective identification: some clinical aspects'. In E. Bott Spillius (ed.) (1988) *Melanie Klein Today, Volume I: Mainly Theory*. London: Routledge.
Jung, C.G. (1921). *Psychological Types. CW6*. London: Routledge & Kegan Paul.
Jung, C.G. (1928–1930). *Dream Analysis*. NJ: Princeton University Press.
Jung, C.G. (1929). *Problems of Modern Psychotherapy. CW16*. London: Routledge & Kegan Paul.
Jung, C.G. (1934–9). 'Nietzsche's Zarathustra'. In C.G. Jung; J. Jarrett (ed.), *Notes of the Seminars Given in 1934–1939*. London: Routledge & Kegan Paul.
Jung, C.G. (1935). *On the Theory and Practice of Analytical Psychology. The Tavistock Lectures.CW18*. London: Routledge & Kegan Paul.
Jung, C.G. (1946). *The Psychology of the Transference. CW16*. Routledge.
Jung, C.G. (1946). *On the Nature of the Psyche. CW8*. London: Routledge & Kegan Paul.
Jung, C.G. (1956). *Symbols of Transformation. CW5*. London: Routledge & Kegan Paul.
Jung, C.G. (1958). *A Psychologicla View of Conscience. CW10*. London: Routledge & Kegan Paul.
Jung, C.G. (1989). 'Nietzsche's Zarathustra'. In C.G. Jung; J. Jarrett (ed.), *Notes of the Seminars Given in 1934–1939*. London: Routledge.
Klein, M. (1946). 'Notes on some schizoid mechanisms'. *International Journal of Psycho-Analysis*, 27, 99–110.
Kradin, R. L. (2011). 'Psychosomatic disorders: the canalization of mind into matter'. *Journal of Analytical Psychology*, 56, 37–55.
Lemma, A. (2015). *Minding the Body: the Body in Psychoanalysis and Beyond*. London: Routledge.
Lombardi, R. and Pola, M. (2010). 'The body, adolescence, and psychosis'. *International Journal of Psychoanalysis*, 91(6), 1419–44.
López-Pedraza, R. (1977). *Hermes and his Children*. Zürich: Spring Publications.
Martini, S. (2016). 'Embodying analysis: the body and the therapeutic process'. *Journal of Analytical Psychology*, 61(1), 5–23.
McDougall, J. (1989). *Theatres of the Body: A Psychoanalytic Approach to Psychosomatic Illness*. London: Free Association Books.
Meltzer, D. (1967). *The Psycho-Analytical Process*. London: Heinemann.
Meltzer, D. (1992). *The Claustrum*. London: Karnac Books.
Modell, A. (1990). *Other Times, Other Realities: Toward a Theory of Psychoanalytic Treatment*. Cambridge, MA: Harvard University Press.
Neumann, E. (1949). *The Place of Creation*. Princeton, NJ: Princeton University Press.
Newton, K. (1965). 'Mediation of the image of infant-mother togetherness'. *Journal of Analytical Psychology*, 10(2), 151–62.
Ogden, T. (1989). *The Primitive Edge of Experience*. Oxford: Jason Aronson.

Ogden, T. (1994). 'On projective identification'. *International Journal of Psycho-Analysis*, 60, 357–373.

Redfearn, J. (2000). 'Possible psychosomatic hazards to the therapist: patients as selfobjects'. *Journal of Analytical Psychology*, 45, 177–94.

Rosenfeld, H. (1971). 'Contribution to the psychology of psychotic states'. In E. Bott Spillius (ed.) (1988) *Melanie Klein Today, Volume I: Mainly Theory*, pp. 117–37. London: Routledge.

Samuels, A. (1985). 'Countertransference, the "Mundus Imaginalis" and a research project'. *Journal of Analytical Psychology*, 30(1), 47–71.

Samuels, A. (2013). 'Countertransference, the imaginal world, and the Politics of the Sublime'. The Jung Page (accessed 30 January 2022) www.cgjungpage.org.

Schwartz-Salant, N. (1982). *Narcissism and Character Transformation: The Psychology of Narcissistic Character Disorders*. Wilmette, IL: Chiron Publications.

Schwartz-Salant, N. (1989). *The Borderline Personality: Vision and Healing*. Wilmette, IL: Chiron Publications.

Schwartz-Salant, N. (1991). 'Vision, interpretation and interaction field'. *Journal of Analytical Psychology*, 3(36), 334–65.

Schwartz-Salant, N. and Stein, M. (1984). *Transference Countertransference*. Wilmette, IL: Chiron Publications.

Schwartz-Salant, N. and Stein, M. (1986). *The Body in Analysis*. Wilmette, IL: Chiron Publications.

Sidoli, M. (2000). *When the Body Speaks: the Archetypes in the Body*. London: Routledge.

Stern, D.N., Sander, L.W., Nahum, J.P., Harrison, A.M., Lyons-Ruth, K., Morgan, A.C., Bruschweilerstern, N. and Tronick, E.Z. (1998). 'Non-interpretative mechanisms in psychoanalytic therapy. The "something more" than interpretation'. *The International Journal of Psychoanalysis*, 79, 903–21.

Stone, M. (2006). 'The analyst's body as tuning fork: embodied resonance in countertransference'. *Journal of Analytical Psychology*, 51, 109–24.

Waska R. (2014). 'Modern Kleinian therapy, Jung's paticipation mystique, and the projective identification process'. In M. Winborn (ed.) (2014) *Shared Realities: Participation Mystique and Beyond*. Skiatook: Fisher King Press.

West, M. (2014). 'Trauma, participation mystique, projective identification and analytical attitude'. In M. Winborn (ed.), (2014) *Shared Realities: Participation mystique and beyond*. Skiatook: Fisher King Press.

Wiener, J. (1994). 'Looking out and looking in.' *Journal of Analytical Psychology*, 39(3), 331–50.

Wiener, J. (2004) *Transference and countertransference: contemporary perspective*. In Cambray, J.; Carter L., ed. (2004) Analytical Psychology. Contenporary Perspectives in Jungian Analysis. Hove: Brunner-Routledge.

Winborn, M. (ed.) (2014). *Shared Realities. Participation Mystique and Beyond*. Skiatook: Fisher King Press.

Wright, S. (2020). 'Analytical attitude – focus or embodiment? Subtle communications in the tranference/countertransference relationship'. *Journal of Analytical Psychology*, 65(3), 538–57.

Chapter 7

American Psychiatric Association. (2013). *Diagnostic and Statistical Manual of Mental Disorders*, 5th ed. Arlington, VA: American Psychiatric Publishing.

Arcelus, J., Mitchell, A.J., Wales, J. and Nielsen, S. (2011). 'Mortality rates in patients with anorexia nervosa and other eating disorders'. *Archives of General Psychiatry*, 68(7), 724–31.

Berenbaum, H. (1996). 'Childhood abuse, alexithymia and personality disorder'. *Journal of Psychosomatic Research*, 41(6), 585–95.

Bick, E. (1968). 'The experience of the skin in early object-relations'. *International Journal of Psychoanalysis*, 49(2–3), 484–6.

Bion, W.R. (1962). 'A theory of thinking'. In *Second Thoughts*, pp. 110–19. London: Karnac, 1984.

Botella, C. and Botella, S. (2005). *The Work of Psychic Figurability*. New York: Brunner/Routledge.

Bromberg, P. (1998). *Standing in the Spaces: Essays on Clinical Process, Trauma, and Dissociation*. Hillsdale, NJ: Analytic Press.

Bromberg, P. (2006). *Awakening the Dreamer: Clinical Journeys*. Hillsdale, NJ: Analytic Press.

Bromberg, P. (2011). *The Shadow of the Tsunami and the Growth of the Relational Mind*. New York: Routledge.

Brown, L.J. (2019). 'Trauma and representation'. *International Journal of Psychoanalysis*, 100(6), 1154–70.

Bruch, H. (1962). 'Perceptual and conceptual disturbances in anorexia nervosa'. *Psychosomatic Medicine*, 24, 187–94.

Bruch, H. (1971). 'Anorexia nervosa in the male'. *Psychosomatic Medicine*, 35(1), 31–47. https://doi.org/10.1097/00006842-197101000-00002 (Accessed 30 January 2022).

Bruch, H. (1973). *Eating Disorders: Obesity, Anorexia Nervosa, and the Person Within*. New York: Basic Books.

Bruch, H. (1978). *The Golden Cage*. Cambridge, MA: Harvard University Press.

Caparrotta, L. and Ghaffari, K. (2006). 'A historical overview of the psychodynamic contributions to the understanding of eating disorders'. *Psychoanalytic Psychotherapy*, 20(3), 175–96.

Chasseguet-Smirgel, J. (1993). 'Eating disorders and femininity: Some reflections on adult cases that presented an eating disorder during adolescence'. *Canadian Journal of Psychoanalysis*, 1(1), 101–12.

Chasseguet-Smirgel, J. (1995). 'Auto-sadism, eating disorders, and femininity: Based on case studies of adult women who experienced eating disorders as adolescents'. In M.A.F. Hanly (ed.), *Essential papers on masochism*. New York: New York University Press.

Craig, A.D. (2004). 'Human feelings: Why are some more aware than others?' *Trends in Cognitive Sciences*, 8, 239–41. doi:10.1016/j.tics.2004.04.004 (Accessed 30 January 2022)

De Berardis, D. et al. (2007). 'Alexithymia and its relationships with body checking and body image in a non-clinical female sample'. *Eating Behaviors*, 8, 296–304.

De Rick, A. and Vanheule, S. (2006). 'The relationship between perceived parenting, adult attachment style and alexithymia in alcoholic inpatients'. *Addictive Behaviors*, 31, 1265–70.

Erikson, E. H. (1993). *Childhood and Society*. W.W. Norton & Company.

Frewen, P.A., Lanius, R.A., Dozois, D.J.A., Neufeld, R.W.J., Pain, C., Hopper, J.W. and Densmore, M. (2008). 'Clinical and neural correlates of alexithymia in PTSD'. *Journal of Abnormal Psychology*, 117, 171–81.

Freud, S. (1920). *Beyond the Pleasure Principle*. S.E., 18. London: Hogarth Press.

Freud, S. (1926). *Inhibitions, Symptoms, and Anxiety*. S.E., 20. London: Hogarth Press.

Garner, D.M. and Garfinkel, P.E. (1980). 'Socio-cultural factors in the development of anorexia nervosa'. *Psychological Medicine*, 10, 647–56.

Garner, D.M., Garfinkel, P.E., Schwartz, D. and Thompson, M. (1980). 'Cultural expectations of thinness in women'. *Psychological Reports*, 47, 483–91.

George, J.B.E. and Franko, D.L. (2010). 'Cultural issues in eating pathology and body image among children and adolescents'. *Journal of Pediatric Psychology*, 35(3), 231–42.

Goldberg, P. (2004). 'Fabricated bodies: A model for the somatic false self'. *International Journal of Psycho-Analysis*, 85, 823–40.

Goodsitt, A. (1997). 'Eating disorders: A self-psychological perspective'. In D.M. Garner and P.E. Garfinkel (eds.), *Handbook of Treatment for Eating Disorders*, 2nd edn. New York: The Guilford Press.

Green, A. (1975). 'The analyst, symbolization, and the absence in the analytic setting'. *International Journal of Psychoanalysis*, 56, 1–22.

Khan, M.M.R. (1963). 'The concept of cumulative trauma'. *Psychoanalytic Study of the Child*, 18, 286–306.

Krystal, H. (1968). *Massive Psychic Trauma*. New York: International Universities Press.

Krystal, H. and Raskin, H. (1970). *Drug Dependence*. Detroit: Wayne State University Press.

Lecours, S. and Bouchard, M-A. (1997). 'Dimensions of mentalisation: Outlining levels of psychic transformation'. *International Journal of Psycho-Analysis*, 78, 855–75.

Lock, J. and Le Grange, D. (2015). *Treatment Manual for Anorexia Nervosa: A Family-based Approach*. Guilford Publications.

Matte-Blanco, I. (1988). *Feeling, Thinking, Being*. Abingdon: Routledge.

Mickalide, A.D. (1990). 'Sociocultural factors influencing weight among males'. In A. Andersen (ed.) *Males with Eating Disorders*, pp. 30–9. Brunner/Mazel.

Miller, S.P., Redlich, A.D. and Steiner, H. (2003). 'The stress response in anorexia nervosa'. *Child Psychiatry and Human Development*, 33, 295–306. doi:10.1023/A:1023036329399 (Accessed 30 January 2022).

Mitchell, J.E. and Crow, S. (2006). 'Medical complications in anorexia nervosa and bulimia nervosa'. *Current Opinion in Psychiatry*, 19, 438–43. doi:10.1097/01.yco.0000228768.79097.3e (Accessed 30 January 2022).

Mond, J.M., Mitchison, D. and Hay, P. (2014). 'Prevalence and implications of eating disordered behavior in men'. In L. Cohn and R. Lemberg (eds.), *Current Findings on Males with Eating Disorders*. Philadelphia, PA: Routledge.

Montebarocci, O., Codispoti, M., Baldaro, B. and Rossi, N. (2004). 'Adult attachment style and alexithymia'. *Personality and Individual Differences*, 36(3), 499–507.

Moulton, R. (1942). 'A psychosomatic study of anorexia nervosa including the use of vaginal smears'. *Psychosomatic Medicine*, 4, 62–74.

Nemiah, J.C. (1977). 'Alexithymia: Theoretical considerations'. *Psychotherapy and Psychosomatics*, 28(1–4), 199–206.

Nemiah, J.C. (1984). 'The psychodynamic view of anxiety'. In R.O. Pasnau (ed.), *Diagnosis and Treatment of Anxiety Disorders*, pp. 117–37. Washington, DC: American Psychiatric Press.

Nowakowski, M.E., McFarlane, T. and Cassin, S. (2013). 'Alexithymia and eating disorders: A critical review of the literature'. *Journal of Eating Disorders*, 1(1), 2.

Orbach, S. (1986). *Hunger Strike*. [Reprinted: London: Karnac, 2005].

Orbach, S. (2002). 'The true self and the false self'. In B. Kahr (ed.), *The Legacy of Winnicott: Essays on Infant and Child Mental Health*. London: Karnac.

Orbach, S. (2009). *Bodies*. New York: Picador.

Paivio, S.C. and McCulloch, C.R. (2004). 'Alexithymia as a mediator between childhood trauma and self-injurious behaviors'. *Child Abuse and Neglect*, 28, 339–54.

Petrucelli, J. (2015). '"My body is a cage": Interfacing interpersonal neurobiology, attachment, affect regulation, self-regulation, and the regulation of relatedness in treatment with patients with eating disorders'. In J. Petrucelli (ed.) *Body-states: Interpersonal and Relational Perspectives on the Treatment of Eating Disorders*. New York: Routledge.

Pine, F. (1983). 'The development of ego apparatus and drive – a schematic view'. *Contemporary Psychoanalysis*, 19, 238–47.

Ridout, N., Thom, C. and Wallis, D.J. (2010). 'Emotion recognition and alexithymia in females with non-clinical disordered eating'. *Eating Behaviors* 11, 1–5.

Rowland, C.V. (1970). 'Anorexia nervosa: A survey of the literature and review of 30 cases'. *International Psychiatric Clinics*, 7, 37–137.

Scheidt, C.E., Waller, E., Schnock, C., Becker-Stoll, F., Zimmerman, P., Lücking, C.H. and Wirsching, M. (1999). 'Alexithymia and attachment representation in idiopathic spasmodic torticollis'. *Journal of Nervous and Mental Disease* 187, 47–52.

Shabad, P. (1993). 'Repetition and incomplete mourning: The intergenerational transmission of traumatic themes'. *Psychoanalytic Psychology*, 10(1), 61–75.

Sifneos, P.E. (1973). 'The prevalence of "alexithymic" characteristics in psychosomatic patients. *Psychotherapy and Psychosomatics*, 22, 255–62.

Smink, F. E., van Hoeken, D. and Hoek, H.W. (2012). 'Epidemiology of eating disorders: Incidence, prevalence and mortality rates'. *Current Psychiatry Reports*, 14(4), 406–14.

Steinhausen, H-C. (2009). 'Outcome of eating disorders'. *Child and Adolescent Psychiatric Clinics of North America*, 18(1) 225–42.

Stice, E., Schupak-Neuberg, K., Shaw, H.E. and Stein, R.I. (1994). 'Relation of media exposure to eating disorder symptomatology: An examination of mediating mechanisms'. *Journal of Abnormal Psychology*, 103, 836–40.

Taylor, G.J. (2004). 'Alexithymia: 25 years of theory and research'. In I. Nyklek, L. Temoshok and A. Vingerhoets (eds.), *Emotion Expression and Health: Advances in Theory, Assessment and Clinical Applications*, pp. 137–53. New York: Brunner-Routledge.

Taylor, G.J. and Bagby, R.M. (2013). 'Psychoanalysis and empirical research: The example of alexithymia'. *Journal of the American Psychoanalytic Association*, 61(1), 99–133.

Troisi, A., D'Argenio, A., Peracchio, F. and Petti, P. (2001). 'Insecure attachment and alexithymia in young men with mood symptoms'. *Journal of Nervous and Mental Disease*, 189, 311–16.

Waller, J.V., Kaufman, M.R. and Deutsch, F. (1940). 'Anorexia nervosa: Psychosomatic entity'. *Psychosomatic Medicine*, 2, 3–16.

Wang, T., Hung, C.C. and Randall, D.J. (2006). 'The comparative physiology of food deprivation: From feast to famine'. *Annual Review of Physiology*, 68(1), 223–51. DOI:10.1146/annurev.physiol.68.040104.105739 (Accessed 30 January 2022).

Westwood, H., Kerr-Gaffney, J., Stahl, D. and Tchanturia, K. (2017). 'Alexithymia in eating disorders: Systematic review and meta-analyses of studies using the Toronto Alexithymia Scale'. *Journal of Psychosomatic Research*, 99, 66–81.

Williams, G. (1997). 'Reflections on some dynamics of eating disorders: "No entry" defenses and foreign bodies'. *International Journal of Psychoanalysis*, 78(5), 927–41.

Winnicott, D.W. (1974). 'Fear of breakdown'. *International Review of Psycho-analysis*, 1, 103–107.

Wooldridge, T. (2014). 'The enigma of ana: A psychoanalytic exploration of pro-ana forums'. *The Journal of Infant, Child, and Adolescent Psychotherapy*, 13(2).

Wooldridge, T. (2016). *Understanding Anorexia Nervosa in Males: An Integrative Approach*. New York: Routledge.

Wooldridge, T. (2018). 'The entropic body: Primitive anxieties and secondary skin formation in anorexia nervosa', *Psychoanalytic Dialogues*, 28(2), 189–202. DOI: 10.1080/10481885.2018.1432949 (Accessed 30 January 2022).

Wooldridge, T. (submitted). 'Anorexia nervosa, psychic death, and the subjugation of need'.
Wooldridge, T. (in press a). 'The paternal function in anorexia nervosa'. *Journal of the American Psychoanalytic Association*.
Wooldridge, T. (in press b). 'Abjection, traumatic themes and alexithymia in anorexia nervosa'. *Contemporary Psychoanalysis*.
Wooldridge, T. and Lytle, P. (2012). 'An overview of anorexia nervosa in adolescent males'. *Eating Disorders: The Journal of Treatment and Prevention*, 20(5), 368–78.
Zerbe, K.J. (1993). *The Body Betrayed: Women, Eating Disorders, and Treatment*. Washington, DC: American Psychiatric Press.
Zlotnick, C., Mattia, J.I. and Zimmerman, M. (2001). 'The relationship between posttraumatic stress disorder, childhood trauma and alexithymia in an outpatient sample'. *Journal of Traumatic Stress* 14, 177–88.

Chapter 8

Aisenstein, M. and de Aisemberg, E.R. (eds.), (2010). *Psychosomatics Today: A Psychoanalytic Perspective*. London: Karnac.
Alvarez, A. (1992). *Live Company: Psychoanalytic Psychotherapy with Autistic, Borderline, Deprived and Abused Children*. London: Routledge.
Alvarez, A. (2012). *The Thinking Heart: Three Levels Of Psychoanalytic Therapy with Disturbed Children*. London: Routledge.
Anzieu, D. (1990). *A Skin for Thought: Interviews with Gilbert Tarrab*. London: Karnac.
Anzieu, D. (2016). *The Skin-Ego*. (N. Segal trans.). London: Routledge.
Bion, W.R. (1970). *Attention and Interpretation*. London: Karnac.
Bollas, C. (1987). *The Shadow of the Object: Psychoanalysis of the Unthought Known*. New York: Columbia University Press.
Bollas, C. (1992). *Being a Character: Psychoanalysis and Self Experience*. New York: Hill and Wang.
Brady, M.T. (2016). *The Body in Adolescence: Psychic Isolation and Physical Symptoms*. London: Routledge.
Bruner, J.S. (1966). On cognitive growth. In J.S. Bruner (Ed.), *Studies in Cognitive Growth*, 1-67. New York: Wiley.
Bucci, W. (1997). 'Symptoms and symbols: A multiple code theory of somatization'. *Psychoanalytic Inquiry*, 17, 151–72.
Bucci, W. (2001). Pathways of emotional communication. *Psychoanalytic Inquiry*, 21: 40-70.
Bucci, W. (2021). *Emotional Communication and Therapeutic Change: Understanding Psychotherapy Through Multiple Code Theory*. London: Routledge.

Caper, R. (1999). *A Mind of One's Own: A Kleinian View of Self and Object*. London: Routledge.
Cornell, W.F. (2008). 'Self in action: The bodily basis of self-organization'. In, F.S. Anderson (ed.), *Bodies in Treatment: The Unspoken Dimension*, pp. 29–50. New York: The Analytic Press.
Cornell, W.F. (2011). 'SAMBA, TANGO, PUNK: Reflections on Steven Knoblauch's "Contextualizing attunement within a polyrhythmic weave: The psychoanalytic samba"'. *Psychoanalytic Dialogues*, 21(4), 428–36.
Cornell, W.F. (2015). *Somatic Experience in Psychoanalysis and Psychotherapy: In the Expressive Language of the Living*. New York: Routledge.
Cornell, W.F. (2016). 'The analyst's body at work: Utilizing touch and sensory experience in psychoanalytic psychotherapies'. *Psychoanalytic Perspectives*, 13, 168–85.
Cornell, W.F. (2019a). '"My body is unhappy": Somatic foundation of script and script protocol'. In *At the Interface of Transactional Analysis, Psychoanalysis, and Body Psychotherapy*, pp. 104–117. London: Routledge.
Cornell, W.F. (2019b). *At the Interface of Transactional Analysis, Psychoanalysis, and Body Psychotherapy: Clinical and Theoretical Perspectives*. London: Routledge.
De Masi, F. (2009). *Vulnerability to Psychosis: A Psychoanalytic Study of the Nature and Therapy of the Psychotic State*. London: Karnac.
Diem-Wille, G. (2021). *Psychoanalytic Perspectives on Puberty and Adolescence: The Inner World of Teenagers and their Parents*. London: Routledge.
Ferrari, A.B. (2004). *From the Eclipse of the Body to the Dawn of Thought*. London: Free Association Books.
Freud, S. (1917/1963). 'Introductory Lectures on Psycho-Analysis: (Part III)'. *The Standard Edition of the Complete Psychological Works of Sigmund Freud*. Volume 16: (1916–1917). London: The Hogarth Press.
Garfield, D.A.S. (2009). *Unbearable Affect: A Guide to the Psychotherapy of Psychosis*. London: Karnac.
Gedo, J.E. (1997). 'The primitive edge, communication, and the language of the body'. *Psychoanalytic Inquiry*, 17, 192–203.
Goldberg, P. (2004). 'Fabricated bodies: A model for the somatic false self'. *International Journal of Psychoanalysis*, 85, 823–40.
Goldberg, P. (2020). 'Body-mind dissociation, altered states, and alter worlds'. *Journal of the American Psychoanalytic Association*, 68, 769–805.
Green, A. (1986). *On Private Madness*. Madison, CT: International Universities Press, Inc.
Laplanche, J. and Pontalis, J-B. (1973). *The Language of Psycho-Analysis*. New York: W.W. Norton & Company.
Lemma, A. (2009). 'Being seen or watched? A psychoanalytic perspective on body dysmorphia'. *International Journal of Psychoanalysis*, 90, 753–71.
Lombardi, R. (2002). 'Primitive mental states and the body: A personal view of Armando B. Ferrari's concrete original object'. *International Journal of Psychoanalysis*, 83, 363–81.

Lombardi, R. (2007). 'Shame in relation to the body, sex, and death: A clinical exploration of the psychotic levels of shame'. *Psychoanalytic Dialogues*, 17, 385-99.

Lombardi, R. (2016). 'Working at the frontiers of nothingness: Homicidal transference, fear of death, and the body'. *Psychoanalytic Psychology*, 33, 80-103.

Lombardi, R. and Pola, M. (2010). 'The body, adolescence, and psychosis'. *The International Journal of Psychoanalysis*, 91, 1419-44.

Lombardi, R., Rinaldi, L., and Thanpulos, S. (2019). *Psychoanalysis of the Psychoses: Current Developments in Theory and Practice*. London: Routledge.

Mitrani, J.L. (1996). *A Framework for the Imaginary: Clinical Explorations in Primitive States of Being*. Northvale, NJ: Jason Aronson Inc.

Mitrani, J.L. (2007). 'Body-centered protections in adolescence: An extension of the work of Frances Tustin'. *International Journal of Psychoanalysis*, 88, 1153-69.

Montemayor, R. (2019). *Sexuality in Adolescence and Emerging Adulthood*. New York: The Guilford Press.

Ogden, T.H. (1989). *The Primitive Edge of Experience*. Northvale, NJ: Jason Aronson Inc.

Orbach, S. (1986). *Hunger Strike*. [Reprinted: London: Karnac, 2005].

Orbach, S. (2002). 'The true self and the false self'. In B. Kahr (ed.), *The Legacy of Winnicott: Essays on Infant and Child Mental Health*. London: Karnac.

Orbach, S. (2009). *Bodies*. New York: Picador.

Piaget, J. (1950). *The Psychology of Intelligence*. London: Routledge & Kegan Paul.

Quinodoz, D. (2003). *Words that Touch: A Psychoanalyst Learns to Speak*. London: Karnac.

Reich, W. (1949). *Character Analysis*. New York: Orgone Institute Press.

Roussillon, R. (2011). *Primitive Agony and Symbolization*. London: Karnac.

Semrad, E. and Van Buskirk, D. (1969). *Teaching Psychotherapy of Psychotic Clients*. New York: Grune and Stratton.

Tustin, F. (1986). *Autistic Barriers in Neurotic Patients*. New Haven, CT: Yale University Press.

Williams, P. (2010). *Invasive Objects: Minds Under Siege*. New York: Routledge.

Winnicott, D.W. (1950/1992). Aggression in relation to emotional development. *Through Paediatrics to Psychoanalysis: Collected Papers*, 204-218. London: Karnac.

Winnicott, D.W. (1964/1989). 'Psycho-somatic illness in its positive and negative aspects'. In C. Winnicott, R. Shepard and M. Davis (eds.), *Psychoanalytic Explorations*, pp. 103-44. Cambridge, MA: Harvard University Press.

Yarom, N. (2015). *Psychic Threats and Somatic Shelters: Attuning to the Body in Contemporary Psychoanalytic Dialogue*. London: Routledge.

Chapter 9

Antliff, M. and Leighten, P. (2003). 'Primitive'. In: R. S. Nelson and R. Shiff (eds.), *Critical Terms for Art History*, pp. 217–32. Chicago: The University of Chicago Press.
Beckett, S. (1964). *How It Is*. London: John Calder.
Boas, F. (1911). *The Mind of Primitive Man*. New York: The Macmillan Company.
Bollas, C. (1987). *Shadow of the Object: Psychoanalysis of the Unthought Known*. London: Free Association Books.
Eekhof, J.K. (2019). *Trauma and Primitive Mental States: An Object Relations Perspective*. Abingdon: Routledge.
Fairbairn, W.R.D. (1952). *Psychoanalytic Studies of the Personality*. London: Tavistock.
Freud, S. (1912–13). *Totem and Taboo. S.E., 13*. London: Hogarth.
Freud, S. (1920). *Beyond the pleasure principle. S.E., 18*. London: Hogarth.
Korff-Sausse, S. (1999). 'A psychoanalytical approach to mental handicap'. In J. De Groeff and E. Heinemann (eds.), *Psychoanalysis and Mental Handicap*, pp. 173–88. London: Free Association Books.
Kovel, J. (1988). *White Racism: A Psychohistory*. London: Free Association Books.
Linington, M. (2009). 'Enduring horror: Psychotherapy with monsters'. *Attachment: New Directions in Relational Psychoanalysis and Psychotherapy*, 3, 53–70.
McCluskey, U. (2005). *To Be Met as a Person*. London: Karnac.
McCluskey, U. and O'Toole, M. (2020). *Transference and Countertransference from an Attachment Perspective: A Guide for Professional Caregivers*. London: Routledge.
Orbach, S. (2009). *Bodies*. London: Profile Books.
Pessoa, F. (1991). *The Book of Disquiet*. A. MacAdam (trans.). Boston: Pantheon Books.
Searles, H. (1979). *Countertransference and Related Subjects*. Madison, WI: International Universities Press.
Shane, M., Shane, E. and Gales, M. (1997). *Intimate Attachments*. London: The Guildford Press.
Shakespeare, W. (1623/1923). *The Tempest*. London: Collins Press.
Sinason, V. (1992). *Mental Handicap and the Human Condition*. London: Free Association Books.
Sullivan, H.S. (1953). *The Interpersonal Theory of Psychiatry*. New York: W.W. Norton & Company.
Van Buren, J. and Alhanti, S. (eds.), (2010). *Primitive Mental States: A Psychoanalytic Exploration of the Origins of Meaning*. New York: Routledge.
Van der Hart, O., Nijenhuis, R.S.E. and Steele, K. (2006). *The Haunted Self: Structural Dissociation and the Treatment of Chronic Traumatisation*. New York: W.W. Norton & Company.
Winnicott, D.W. (1971). 'Mirror-role of mother and family in child development'. In D.W. Winnicott, *Playing and Reality*, pp. 111–18. London: Tavistock.

Index

abandonment 6, 8, 17, 70, 105, 115, 135, 137, 184–185, 189, 190
Abraham, K. 4, 6, 44
abuse
   adolescence/relational history 104
   mother and infant 122–123
   olfactory communication 89–91
   sexual trauma 10, 27, 33, 44–45, 75–76, 90–91, 152
adolescence
   and abuse 104
   body 169, 170, 178
   eating disorders 141–142, 143, 154–155
   emergent sexuality 162–164
adoption 103–104, 112, 116, 184
affect/body 161–162, 172–173
alexithymia 146–153
anal/genital intrusion 58, 137–138
'analyst-centred interpretations' 108–109
analytic/therapeutic dyad 121
Anna O (Pappenheim) xxii, 2
annihilation anxiety 146–149, 150, 155, 158
anorexia nervosa 141–155
Anthony, E. J. 43
anti-libidinal ego/internal saboteur 192
anti-Semitism 85
anxiety
   consulting rooms 2, 72–73, 98
   'dissolution of boundedness' 127
   drawings of 32–38
   and dread 104–105
   entropic body 141–144, 146–149, 150, 151, 154
   fear of dying 104–105
Anzieu, D. 81, 92, 100–101, 160
Apparently Normal Person (ANP) 192
aristocracy 86–87
art of health/smelliness 80–82
asylum/community societal structuring 82
attachment 54, 59, 71, 100, 105, 107, 112, 117, 152, 183, 185, 191
'autistic-contiguous' modes (Ogden) 127, 160

babies
   in context of trauma 51
   fear of dying 104–105
   olfactory communication 81–82
   oral phase of psychosexual development 142–143
'bad air'/miasma theory 86–88
baptisms 85
Barrows, P. 44
Beckett, S. 191
bedwetting 5
bereavement 70–71, 73–74
   counselling 63–64, 73–74
   see also grief
beta-endorphins and self-harm 66–67
'betrayal by the body'/sexual abuse 90–91
Bick, E. 32, 46, 100, 127, 146, 149–151
Bion, W.R. 25, 45–46, 82, 94, 100–105, 121, 144, 151, 158
   alexithymia 153
   baby's fear of dying 104–105
   mother and rêverie 120–121
   'nameless dread' 94, 104–105
   'problem of groupishness' 82
   projective identification 123
   psychical container 100–101
bipolar disorder 184–185
biting 63–64
blame 67
bodily ego 88, 93
bodily invasion 28–29
   see also sexual trauma
body babblings/borderline of Hermes 130–134
body modification in adult life 90
body odour 79, 84, 99–118
   human evolution 83–84

225

olfactory communication 79–98
  see also smell
Bollas, C. 173–175, 182
borderline of Hermes (López-Pedraza) 130–134
borderline personality disorder 110
bourgeoisie 86–87
Brady, M.T. 168–169
Breuer, J. 2
Brill, A. 6–7
British Sign Language 71–72
Bromberg, P. 143
Brown, L.J. 105
Bruch, H. 143
Bucci, W. 161, 175–176

'Cabbage Liberation' (poem) 60
Caper, R. 159
caregivers
  annihilation/signal anxiety 146–149
  Coniunctio 134–138
  death and bereavement 70–71, 73–74
  neglect 170–171
  Oedipal sexuality 44–45, 103–104, 114–115, 134
  primordial stage of the mother–child relationship 135
  and rêverie 120–121
  skin-ego (Anzieu) 160–161
  violence toward infant 122–123
Carvalho, R. 137
character analysis 172–173
Chasseguet-Smirgel, J. 144
Chestnut Lodge sanatorium, Rockville 7–8
Child and Adolescent Mental Health Service (CAMHS) 71
children
  Coniunctio 134–138
  mistreatment 89
  neglect 88, 89, 152, 170–171
  psychotherapy training 51
  psychotic 43–44
  sexual trauma 10, 33, 44–45, 75–76, 90–91, 152
  social countertransference 94–95
  see also infants
China and toilet paper 54

Christian baptisms 85
'civilized' society (hygiene) 80–82, 84
Clark, G. 122–123
classical psychoanalysis and psychotherapy 46–47
  see also Freud
classism and olfactory communication 86–87
claustrophobia 94, 102–103
cleanliness 1
'communicate' origins 93
compulsive spitting 13–42
confidentiality 68
Coniunctio 134–138
Connolly, A. 122
consciousness 121–122
consulting rooms for intellectual disability 71–77
consumption of urine/faeces 4, 59
containment of self 45, 94–95
Corbett, A. 75–76
Corbin, H. 121
counselling 63–64, 73–74
countertransference 29–30
  awareness of 69–70
  embodied 130–134
  hate in (Winnicott) 106, 109
  hygiene 82
  olfactory communication 79, 91, 97
  social countertransference 82, 94–95, 94–96
  'syntonic countertransference' 120–121
  unconscious somatic communication 119–140
  Winnicott 106, 109
Covid-19 pandemic 57–58, 80
crayons and drawing 32–38
cult abuse 59

De Masi, F. 159
De Rienzo, A. 131
death 70–71
  baby's fear of dying 104–105
  death/death drive 141–142, 149
  social death 91
denial 142–143
destruction of the sense of self 122–123

dirt 79, 82, 83, 89, 94–95, 174–175, 177
'disposable' people in Greek culture 55–57
dissociation 136–138
dissociative identity disorder (DID) 191–196
'dissolution of boundedness' 127
distress, olfactory communication 81–82
'disturbances in vitality' (Wiener) 122
Douglas, M. 82, 83
Down's syndrome 55–57, 183–191
drawing 32–38
dread 94, 104–105
 see also anxiety
dreaming 108–109, 110–112, 116–117
'dreaming mind' (Wright) 131
drug dependence 152

eating disorders 141–146
Eder, M.D. 6
ego
 anorexia nervosa 142–143, 145–146
 anti-libidinal ego/internal saboteur 192
 olfactory communication 88
 oral phase of psychosexual development 142–143
 skin-ego (Anzieu) 100–101, 160–161
 subtle body 130–131
Eitingon, M. 5
ejaculation see spitting
elderly people 59–60
Elmhirst, S.I. 45
embodied countertransference
 body babblings/borderline of Hermes 130–134
 Coniunctio 134–138
 Nigredo 125–130
 as 'organ of information' 120–124
 and unconscious somatic communication 119–140
emotional maturity 178–179
emotional neglect 152
 see also neglect
empirical studies on alexithymia 152
endorphins and self-harm 66–67
entropic body 141–155
 alexithymia 146, 151–153
 annihilation anxiety 146–149

signal anxiety 146–149
environment
 intellectual disability and self-harm 67
 see also caregivers
erotic arousal through vomiting 8
Eulert-Fuchs, D. 130
European Commission 55
European cultural knowledge about smell 85–86
evolution 83–84
excretory organs 83–84
existential emptiness/helplessness 122
eye-poking 63–64

'fabricated bodies' 163–164, 173
faeces 4–8, 51–54, 58
Fairbairn, W.R.D. 95, 96, 192
false bodies 163–164, 173
false body 141, 146, 163, 173
family-based therapy (FBT) 141–142
FBT see family-based therapy
fear of dying 104–105
Ferro, A. 125
first World War 88
foetor Judaicus (innate stench of the Jew) 85
Fordham, M. 120–121
Freud, A. 5
Freud, J. 5
Freud, S. 2–6, 44, 83–84
 annihilation/signal anxiety 147–148
 eating disorders 142–143
 entropic body 147–148, 149
 melancholy 95–96
 sensate/somatic domains 171–172
 'shell shock' 88
 trauma/traumata/psychotherapy 181
Fromm-Reichmann, F. 7–8
funerals 70–71

Garfield, D.A.S. 170, 172–173
Gayetty, J. 54
Geller, J. 85
genital intrusion 6–7, 21, 58, 137–138
 see also sexual trauma
genitals/excretory organs 83–84
genocidal scapegoating 84–85

germ theory 87–88
Goldberg, P. 163, 173
grief 70–71, 73–74
haematemesis (vomiting of blood) 7
'handicapped smile' concepts 66
'Hate in the Countertransference' (Winnicott) 106, 109
Hodges, S. 70
hostility 27
human evolution 83–84
Hurley, A.D. 72
hygiene 80–82

ID *see* intellectual disability
impotence 122
in corpore inventitur (embodied countertransference) 119–140
incorporation 88
incorporation/possession 136–138
individual/communal societal structuring 82
infantilization 73
infants
   annihilation/signal anxiety 146–149
   entropic body 149–150
   with regard to 'primitive' 159
   rêverie of the mother 120–121
   and skin-ego (Anzieu) 100–101
   violence of mother 122–123
insecure attachment 152
intellectual disability (ID) 13–26, 55–60, 63–78, 183–191
   consulting room 71–77
   definition 64–65
   mental health and trauma 65–66
   network 67–70
   self-harm 63, 66–67
   Tavistock Clinic 14–42, 121
   therapeutic challenges 70–71
internalizing anxiety/internal distress 63–78, 146–149
   see also trauma/traumata
interpersonal context and olfactory communication 93–94
interpretation 30–31
'intersubjective unconscious experiences' (Wiener) 131–132

Island of Leros, Greece 55–57

Jenner, M. 84
Jewish communities and social ostracism 85
Jones, E. 2–3, 43
judgment 69–70
Jung, C.G. 3–6
   body babblings/borderline of Hermes 130–131
   'kinship libido' 134–135
   participation mystique 119, 124, 131
   psychoid realm 121
   'reconciliation of opposites' 134–135
   'symbolic homosexuality' 136

Kahr, B. 105
Kettler, A. 85–86
'kinship libido' (Jung) 134–135
Klein, M. 26, 93–94, 100, 114–115, 123
knowing 161–162
Kolvin, I. 55
Kovel, J. 181
Kraeplin, E. 6

language/cognition 161–162
Lanzer, Ernst (Rattenmann/Rat Man) 5
Laplanche, J. 172
learning 161–162
Lemma, A. 90
Levitas, A.S. 72
Lombardi, R. 125, 158, 162–163
loneliness 93–94
López-Pedraza, R. 130–134

McDougall, J. 122–123
Makaton signing 71–72
Marcus Valerius Martialis 1
masturbation 6–7, 21
   see also spitting
maturity 159–160, 178–179
Meltzer, D. 103
Mental Handicap and the Human Condition: New Approaches from the Tavistock 14–15
mental health
   practitioners 3

Index   229

self-harm/intellectual disability 65–66
mephitic other 79, 84–85
'metabolism'/processing of experiences 88
miasma theory 86–88
mind–body relationships 92, 122
    see also splitting
Mitrani, J.L. 100
Modell, A. 122–124
molestation 33
    see also sexual trauma
'moments of meeting' (Stern) 131–132
mother figures
    annihilation/signal anxiety 146–149
    neglect 170–171
    Oedipal sexuality 44–45, 103–104,
        114–115, 134
    primordial stage of the mother–child
        relationship 135
    and rêverie 120–121
    violence toward infant 122–123
motoric system activation 27, 152
    see also anxiety
'Mourning and Melancholia' (Freud) 95–96
mucous 31–32, 44, 51–52
Multiple Code Theory 161–162

Nabokov, V. 99–100
'nameless dread' (Bion) 94, 104–105
Napoleon Bonaparte 84
narcissistic personality disorder 110
nausea 29–31, 126–127, 132, 134
Nazism 57, 85
neglect 88, 89, 152, 170–171
Nemiah, J.C. 152–153
neuroses 171–172
neurotic spitting and psychotic smearing
    9–13
Newton, K. 122–123
NHS consulting room 72
NHS multidisciplinary team 64
NHS service 71
NICE guidelines 89
Nigredo 125–130
non-directive approaches 69–70
non-judgmental attitudes 69–70
non-verbal information 69–70
non-verbal patients and trauma 51–61

'Notes on Some Schizoid Mechanisms'
    (Klein) 123

'object of pity' stereotypes 73
object relating/object usage 110
obsessive compulsive disorder (OCD)
    176–180
odour 99–118
    human evolution 83–84
    olfactory communication 79–98
    see also smell
Oedipal sexuality 44–45, 103–104, 114–115,
    134
Ogden, T. 100, 127, 160–161
olfactory communication 79–98
    abuse 89–91
    applying psychoanalysis 87–88, 94–96
    bodily ego 88
    child mistreatment 89
    classism 86–87
    conceptual and historical territories 83–87
    dirt/disorder 83
    dread 94
    failure of indwelling 92
    interpersonal context 93–94
    Jewish communities 85
    loneliness 93–94
    melancholic object 95–96
    mephitic other79 84–85
    racism 85–86
    repression 83–84
    social countertransference 94–96
omnipotence 138
openness 69–70
oral phase of psychosexual development
    142–143
'organ of information' (Fordham) 120–124
orifices 51–52
'Over and Out' (Nightshift 1995) 55

panic disorders 152
Pappenheim, Bertha 2
paranoid schizophrenia 11–13,123, 134
Parson, J. 70
participation mystique (Jung) 119, 124, 131
'patient-centred interpretations' 108–109
'perceptual systems' (Fordham) 120–124

Perfume: The Story of a Murderer (Süskind) 100
'perpetual children' stereotypes 73
personal hygiene 80–82, 84
pervasive relational trauma 143
'perversions' and smell 83–84
Petrucelli, J. 143
phthisis (tuberculosis of the lungs) 7
physical abuse 152
    see also abuse
physical neglect 152
    see also neglect
Pine, F. 148
Pola, M. 125, 162–163
Pontalis, J.-B. 172
pornography 136–138
possession 136–138
pre-Oedipal sexuality 134
primordial stage of the mother–child relationship 135
private/public societal structuring 82
'problem of groupishness' (Bion) 82
processing of experiences 88
projection 88
projective identification 123–124, 127–128
Proust, M. 99–100
psyche
    and 'organ of information' 120–121
    with regard to 'primitive' 158–160
    secondary to body 157–180
psychic elaboration of emotion 152–153
psychic trauma 152
    see also trauma/traumata
psychical container 100–101
    see also containment of self
psychoanalysis
    body odour 99–118
    ideas of 'symptoms' 81–82
    olfactory communication 87–88
psychogenic vomiting 8
    see also vomiting
psychoid realm 120–121
'psycho-somatic partnership' (Winnicott) 122–123
psychotherapy 69–70, 181–197
psychotic patients 4, 5–8
    children 43–44

defences and role of affect 172–173
neurotic spitting and psychotic smearing 9–13
punishment/blame 67
Purity and Danger (Douglas) 82, 83

Quinodoz, D. 157

Rabelais 54
racism 53–54, 85–86
Rank, O. 5
rape 59
    see also sexual trauma
'reactions to impingement' (Reich) 173
'reconciliation of opposites' (Jung) 134–135
'Redecur'/'talking cure' 2
Reich, W. 172–173, 175–176
relational history/body odour 103–104
religion 85
Remembrance of Things Past (Proust) 99–100
retching 127
    see also vomiting
rêverie
    Coniunctio 134–138
    of the mother 120–121
Riviere, J. 2–3
Rolland, R. 85

sadism/libidinal strivings 44–45
Samuels, A. 121
scapegoating 84–85, 94–95
Schick, A. 8
schizophrenia 11–13, 123, 134
Schwartz-Salant, N. 120–121, 131, 134–135
scratching 63–64, 74–75
'second skin formation' (Bick) 127
'secondary handicap' 17–18
secret/ostentatious societal structuring 82
seizures 184
self-care 80–82
self-denial 142–143
self-esteem/self-cohesion 143
self-harm, intellectual disability 63, 66–67
self-holding 149–150
self-sensation 120–121
'semi-hallucinatory elaboration' (De Rienzo) 131

Semrad, E. 172–173
sensate/somatic domains 171–174
sensate/somatic organization 160–162
'sense of deadness' (Connolly) 122
sense of self 122–123
separation anguish 135
sexual trauma 10, 33, 44–45, 75–76, 90–91, 152
sexuality 134–138, 176–179
  adolescence 162–164
  Oedipal 44–45, 103–104, 114–115, 134
  sensate/somatic domains 171–172
Shakespeare, W. 51
Shared Realities – Participation Mystique and Beyond 124
'shell shock' 88
Sidoli, M. 122–123, 138
Sifneos, P.E. 152
signal anxiety 146–149
Sinason, V. 14–15, 17–18, 29–30, 65–66, 67
skin-ego (Anzieu) 100–101, 160–161
smearing 6–7, 9–13, 14, 58
smell 60–61, 79–98
  human evolution 83–84
  olfactory communication 79–98
  racism 53–54, 85–86
  'smelly' people/art of health 80–82
  The Smell of Slavery (Kettler) 85–86
sneezing 31–32, 44
Socarides, C. 8
social countertransference/olfactory communication 82, 94–96
'social death' 91
social exclusion 80–82, 84–85
somatic communication 119–140
  countertransference 30
  olfactory communication 81–82
  organization 160–162
  separation anguish 135
  unconscious 130–134
Spielrein, S. 3–4
spitting 1–49
  compulsive 13–42
  neurotic spitting and psychotic smearing 9–13
splitting 55–57, 122, 134–135
Stallybrass, P. 86

starvation/anorexia nervosa 141–146
Steiner, J. 108–109
stereotypes 73, 84–85
Stern, D. 131–132
STOMP government campaign 67
Stone, M. 130–131
subtle body 130–131
suffocation and dread 94
  see also claustrophobia
Sullivan, H.S. 183
superego 142–143
Süskind, P. 100
'symbolic homosexuality' (Jung) 136
Symington, N. 68, 70
'syntonic countertransference' 120–121

'talking cure' 2
Tavistock Clinic 14–42, 121
therapeutic dyad 121, 130–131
toddlers 51
  see also children; infants
toileting behaviour 38–40
toilet paper 54
  see also urine/faeces
tolerance/toleration 29, 30–31
touch, wariness of 57–58
transference, awareness of 69–70
trauma/traumata
  alexithymia 152
  anorexia nervosa 141–146
  bodily ego 88
  body odour/psychoanalytic treatment 99–118
  communication of 183–191
  drawing 32–38
  entropic body 143, 149–150
  non-verbal patients 51–61
  psychotherapy 181–197
  'second skin formation' (Bick) 127
  self-harm/intellectual disability 65–66
  sensate/somatic domains 171–172
  sexual trauma 10, 33, 44–45, 75–76, 90–91, 152
  spitting 17, 30, 44–47
Die Traumdeutung (The Interpretation of Dreams) (Freud) 5, 44
Tsiantis, J. 55

tuberculosis 7
Tustin, F. 43–44
unconscious somatic communication 119–140
unfelt feelings 191–196
'unthought known' 182–183
Upton, P. 70
urine/faeces 4–8, 51–54, 58

Van Buskirk, D. 172–173
verbal information 69–70
visceral/motoric system activation 27, 152
   see also anxiety
vomiting 7, 8, 127, 174
Vulnerability to Psychosis (De Masi) 159

wariness of touch 57–58
Weininger, B. 8
well being and hygiene 80–82
West, M. 124
When Mum Died 73
When Somebody Dies 73
White, A. 86

'white heat' 45
Wiener, J. 122, 131–132
Winborn, M. 131
Winnicott, D.W. 45
   body odour/psychoanalytic treatment 106, 109–110
   communicating trauma 191
   dimensions of neglect 89
   entropic body 149–150
   failure of indwelling 92
   'psycho-somatic partnership' 122–123
   sensate/somatic domains 173–174
World War I 88
Wright, S. 127, 131

young adults, eating disorders 141–142
young children 5–6
   see also children; infants

Zarathustra, N. 131
Zerbe, K.J. 144

Karnac Books, founded in 1950 and relaunched in 2020, publishes seminal and contemporary texts on psychotherapy and psychoanalysis. It continues its long tradition of exploring the intricacies of these disciplines, providing space for the best writers on the complexities of the mind.